D0843430

Modern European History

A Garland Series of Outstanding Dissertations

General Editor
William H. McNeill
University of Chicago

Associate Editors

Eastern Europe
Charles Jelavich
Indiana University

Great Britain
Peter Stansky
Stanford University

France
David H. Pinkney
University of Washington

Russia
Barbara Jelavich
Indiana University

Germany
Enno E. Kraehe
University of Virginia

MODERN EUROPEAN HISTORY

Doctors, Bureaucrats, and Public Health in France, 1888–1902

Martha L. Hildreth

Garland Publishing, Inc.
New York and London 1987

Library of Congress Cataloging-in-Publication Data

Hildreth, Martha Lee.
    Doctors, bureaucrats, and public health in France,
1888–1902.

    (Modern European history)
    Bibliography: p.
    1. Trade-unions—Physicians—France—History—
19th century.   2. Physicians—France—Political activity—History—19th century.   3. Medical laws and
legislation—France—History—19th century.   4. Medicine—France—History—19th century.
I. Title.   II. Series.
R728.3.H55   1987   362.1'72'0944   87-7542
ISBN 0-8240-8037-8 (alk. paper)

All volumes in this series are printed on acid-free,
250-year-life paper.

Printed in the United States of America

DOCTORS, BUREAUCRATS AND PUBLIC HEALTH IN FRANCE, 1888-1902

Martha L. Hildreth

To my parents, Leroy and Ila Hildreth

PREFACE

In preparing my Ph.D. dissertation for publication I have taken the opportunity to make some revisions. Most are only grammatical; however, I have reorganized and (I hope) clarified some material. No new material has been added thus the bibliography is somewhat out of date having been compiled in 1982. I have taken the liberty of adding some footnotes which refer the reader to my own more recent work where appropriate.

I would like to acknowledge the invaluable help in manuscript preparation given to me by the Text Processing Center and the Department of Mathematics, University of Nevada, Reno. Text preparation costs were supported in part by the Center for Advanced Studies, College of Arts and Science, University of Nevada, Reno. In the preparation of the tables I was generously assisted by Charles Wetherell of the Laboratory for Historical Research, University of California Riverside. In the course of research I received vital help from the staff of the Archives de la Santé publique, Paris.

During the original preparation of the dissertation, and in the months since, a number of people have read and made helpful comments upon the manuscript. I would like to thank Ken Barkin, Patricia O'Brien, Alan Mitchell, George Weisz, and most particularly, Irwin Wall.

During various stages of my work on this manuscript my family has been a steadfast source of support. I would like to to aknowledge the the help given to me by my parents and the moral support of my sister, Margaret Rhyne, during the long months of research. Lastly, my husband, Bruce Blackadar, has been an ever patient source of support during my more recent revisions of the manuscript. I thank him for his help in proof reading and in formatting the manuscript for printing on a computerized text processing system. Most of all I am grateful for his tolerance while I spent a good deal of a supposed vacation revising the text.

Reno, Nevada
November, 1986

TABLE OF CONTENTS

Preface   iii

Table of Contents   v

List of Figures and Tables   vi

Introduction   1

Chapter   I: French Doctors 1888-1902: A Profession in Crisis   36

Chapter II: The National Public Health Bureaucracy and the   107
              Bacteriological Revolution

Chapter III: The Loi Chevandier   164

Chapter IV: The Creation of a National Medical Assistance   215
              Program

Chapter   V: The Impact of the Medical Assistance Law,   314
              1893-1902

Conclusion   327

Bibliography   335

Appendices   348

LIST OF TABLES AND FIGURES

Figure I-1: Docteurs, Officiers de santé, and Total
Practitioners in France, 1847-1906 ... 82

Figure I-2: Docteurs, Officiers de santé, and Total
Practitioners in France, 1847-1906 ... 84

Table I-1: Practitioners per Population in France,
1847-1906 ... 85

Table I-2: Density of Officiers de santé, Docteurs, and
Total Practitioners by Department in 1896 ... 86

Table I-3: Medical Density in 1881 for Departments
Containing Areas with the Greatest Rates of
Urban Growth in the Nineteenth Century ... 91

Table III-1: Departments with the Greatest Loss of
Officiers de santé, 1866-1896 ... 205

Table IV-1: Functioning of Medical Assistance Under
Different Systems in 1887 ... 255

Table V-1: Functioning of Medical Assistance Under
Different Systems in 1899 ... 313

DOCTORS, BUREAUCRATS AND PUBLIC HEALTH IN FRANCE, 1888-1902

INTRODUCTION

The years 1888-1902 were a crucial period in the creation of a modern medical system in France. Scientific developments, demographic and political concerns sparked an unprecedented period of government action concerning medical care. The nature of the resulting legislation was largely determined by a new medical union movement, promoting the professional goals of private physicians. The effects of these developments were manifold. In this period doctors were given state support which allowed them to dominate medical care as they never had before. A variety of public health services were created and ultimately a basic public health law was passed. A national medical assistance program was created to bring medical care to the rural poor. Finally, a number of new medical institutions evolved, including dispensaries, disinfection services, sanatoriums and medical insurance. Although overshadowed in the standard histories of the Third Republic by the tumultuous political events of the period, the medical developments of 1888-1902 received considerable attention from legislators, bureaucrats and intellectuals of the time. Moreover these medical developments would ultimately have a tremendous impact on the general population. As Eugen Weber has indicated, this period saw the transformation of a disparate, rural, French society into a more homogeneous nation. The medical developments of the era should be included along side the modernization of education and transportation in the constellation of changes which most affected people's everyday lives. [1]

The medical care system which evolved in France during this period combined state services with a liberal, private profession in what has been aptly called the "hybridization" of medical care. [2] The hybrid medical system is of course typical of most modern, capitalist nations, where modern medicine has been accompanied by the professionalization of doctors and their dominance over the practice of medicine.

It is a popularly held notion that professionalization came about in the late nineteenth century as a result of the development and adoption by the medical profession of a unified and effective theory of disease, the germ theory. [3] According to this viewpoint, established doctors were able to rally around the germ theory and use it to support their claims to dominate the practice of medicine and exclude unlicensed practitioners. Physicians' claims were backed by the modern state which began to become interested in improving the health of its citizens by promoting modern medical care. The state thus granted physicians an autonomous position in regulating their own profession and helped them to dominate the whole medical care system. This explanation, however, does not suit the development of modern medicine in France. Some French doctors were professionalized about one hundred years earlier. In addition, the French state took a very active role in medical care as early as the late eighteenth century. [4]

According to Toby Gelfand and David M. Vess, by the end of the eighteenth century, French doctors had developed a very "modern" notion of the status of their occupation as a profession and had achieved some of the major qualities which most sociologists see as characteristic of a profession. [5] Most importantly, they achieved control over medical education and through the law of March 10, 1803. [6] Gelfand also argues that in the late eighteenth and early nineteenth centuries physicians achieved a unified theoretical basis of practice based upon the clinical model developed at the Paris hospitals; however, this contention is contradicted by several other works. [7]

In contrast to Gelfand and Vess, the work of Jacques Léonard, Jean-Pierre Goubert, George Weisz and Matthew Ramsey on the social and economic status of French doctors in the nineteenth century has shown that the average French doctor lived and practiced in a condition which was far from the status of a professional in modern times. [8] Léonard shows that the average doctor occupied a humble place among the French bourgeoisie through most of the nineteenth century. Léonard's work, along with that of Weisz and Ramsey, indicates that doctors struggled economically, rarely enjoyed the medical confidence of their local society, and competed with a wide range of traditional healers and practitioners. Ramsey found that in spite of the legislation of 1803, local officials actually protected illegal practitioners.

Léonard, Goubert, Weisz and Ramsey on one hand and Gelfand and Vess on the other might seem to be talking about two different worlds, and indeed they are. As a number of historians have pointed out, the societies of urban and rural France were worlds apart in the nineteenth century. [9] According to Harvey Mitchell, in the late eighteenth century the French medical world was divided into two exclusive systems: traditional, unlicensed medicine on the one hand, which treated the health problems of rural society and the lower urban classes, and elite physicians on the other, who practiced among the urban bourgeoisie and aristocracy. Mitchell further points out that rather than attempting to destroy traditional medicine, the urban elites tended to believe that the two different kinds of medicine were appropriate for their respective worlds. [10] This left licensed rural practitioners to struggle alone against illegal practitioners without much official support. Medical elites in the cities were not particularly concerned with sharing the benefits of professionalization with their more humble country brothers. [11] In order to understand the professionalization process among French doctors it is crucial to make this distinction between the of urban, academic elites and the average private practitioner of the villages and quartiers.

In the case of French doctors, it is useful to think of professionalization as a concept which originated among the elite physicians in the late eighteenth and early nineteenth century, and then, only much later, became a reality for the average practitioner. How to define the elites is not an easy task. Certainly they would include the members of the Faculty of Medicine and Academy of Medicine in Paris who also dominated the prestigious hospital posts in that city. Also they would include doctors in similar positions in the other faculties of medicine at Bordeaux and Montpellier. In the course of the nineteenth century, some other urban centers also developed medical establishments: Havre, Lyon, Reims, Rennes, Toulouse and Lille. [12] Léonard has also found evidence that there was a group of rural elite doctors in the nineteenth century who achieved status through former academic positions, personal wealth, or bureaucratic posts. [13] These elites enjoyed high prestige and wealth from their academic and bureaucratic positions and were able to attract a profitable clientele from among the haute-bourgeoisie. They did not have to struggle to lure clients away from popular practitioners such as bonesetters and urine readers. Their only competition was among themselves.

The mass of doctors envied the benefits enjoyed by the elites, recognized the benefits of professionalization and aspired to transform their positions into something more like that of the elites. The large number of average practitioners who attended the Medical Congress of 1845 clearly demonstrated these desires. [14] Professional concepts were well known to the mass of practitioners, but until the last two decades of the century they were not able to translate these concepts into reality in their own practices. Until then private practitioners had made periodic and unsuccessful efforts to obtain a revision of the law of 1803 on the practice of medicine in order to increase the severity of the regulations against illegal practitioners and to give all *docteurs* a monopoly over medical practice in their own areas. [15]

The extension of professional status to the lower orders of *docteurs* was greatly aided by the final achievement of a new law on the practice of medicine, passed in 1892. The 1892 law was passed in the midst of the bacteriological revolution; however, the relationship between the scientific developments and the attainment of professional status by the average practitioners was ambiguous. The connection between the establishment of germ theory and the effectiveness of medical techniques cannot be assumed. Neither can physicians be assumed to have welcomed many of the new techniques and practices with the germ theory implied. The role of medical effectiveness in professionalization must be examined more closely. Since René Dubois first raised the issue in 1959, several researchers have maintained that the apparent improvements in health as measured by increased life span, which took place in the nineteenth century, were the result primarily of improvements in diet and quite later in the century, the result of public health measures. The only medical development which may have affected general health before the latter part of the nineteenth century was vaccination against smallpox. [16] As Thomas McKeown has pointed out, this fact has been largely ignored in the traditional literature on the history of medicine which concentrates on scientific developments. Medical historians have made little investigation into when and how these developments actually were put into practice and whether they had any beneficial effects on general health. [17]

What effect did the bacteriological revolution have on medical practice? Léonard remarks that it was the work of Pasteur and Lister which began to improve the economic and social status of the mass of practitioners after 1885. Léonard is careful to note that the *reputation* of official medicine improved as a result of the overwhelming publicity which Pasteur and his theories received after 1885. He does not credit the actual practices of individual doctors as having much impact on health, although he does imply that some doctors may have had a positive impact on health through the massive outpouring of advisory literature which they began to produce for popular consumption in this era. [18] McKeown maintains that effective techniques in medical practice were not developed until the twentieth century. [19] The type of medical changes implied by the development of the germ theory were those which lay in the realm of public health rather than private practice. As this work will show, the governments and bureaucracy of the Third Republic became interested in promoting new public health policies and programs, but private practitioners opposed many of these plans as threats to their status as liberal professionals. Nevertheless, French doctors were able to exploit the favorable reputation created by the work of Pasteur and Lister as well as the health concerns of the state to promote their professional goals.

The relationship of physicians to the state and to society is of course critical in understanding the process of professionalization. Sociologists studying the professions have concentrated their analysis on these issues. Talcott Parsons built his model of professionalization largely upon an analysis of the profession of medicine. Basically, he interpreted the phenomenon of the profession as arising from a sructural need of society. The need, in the case of medicine, was for a body of workers who could be trusted to fulfill a specialized technical function which the layman cannot comprehend or perform. The social body, according to Parsons, confers a monopoly on this body of experts in return for which the profession assures high standards of application of technical expertise, devotion to the interests of society, and honorability. For Parsons, the interests of the patient are the functional norm which define the profession.

Jeffrey Berlant, who also builds his model on the profession of medicine, maintains, contrary to Parson, that "the dominant force defining the profession is the collective interest of physicians which may or may not benefit patients." Berlant further argues that traditionally the medical profession has defined health in terms of the individual; most of the profession has been indifferent or even hostile to many public health activities. Finally, Berlant believes that there is no fundamental distinction between the profession and the world of business. As a pay-for-service activity, the profession of medicine arose as part of the free market economy; it offers a service in exchange for a price, and the service is based upon an unwritten contract between buyer and seller. [20]

In his work focusing on the modern medical profession, Eliot Freidson emphasizes the circumstances of medical practice as crucial in defining the nature of the profession itself. Freidson explains that basically the practice of medicine is an encounter between two individuals, the doctor and the client. The doctor is oriented towards dealing with individual problems, not broader social concerns. In fact, Freidson argues that the profession attracts those individuals who like to avoid broad political and social issues. Thus it creates practitioners who are biased in favor of direct action in a private setting. In other words, the profession attracts those who seek autonomy; therefore the nature of the practice, the one-to-one encounter, is reinforced by the personal orientation of the individuals who are attracted to the profession. For Freidson, individualism is thus the dominant element in the profession; he writes, "contrary to Parson, I would suggest that the practitioner is particularistic *not* universalistic." [21]

Freidson's other valuable insights include his realization that the connection to science is a key in explaining the rise of the profession of medicine. This connection allowed medicine to expand into terrain once held only by law and theology. He argues that as human welfare became secularized, the helping professions arose as service workers to the state. This general phenomenon has also been described by Christopher Lasch and Jacques Donzelot in relation to the history of the family. [22] Freidson concludes, "Medicine's position today is akin to that of religion's yesterday - it has an officially approved monopoly of the right to define health and to treat illness." [23]

Freidson also points out the importance of the formation of a coherent or accepted ideology in enabling a profession to become both cohesive within itself and validated to the outside world. He sees the rise of bacteriological medicine as the crucial event for the professionalization of medicine. Before this, acording to Freidson, physicians were simply a "learned group aspiring toward monopoly." [24]

Finally, Freidson stresses the role of the state in professionalizing medicine. The practice of medicine, he points out, is a consulting profession. It depends upon public obedience to the principle that there is only one group with whom it should consult in the case of illness. The promotion of an ideology is an important factor in assuring such behavior; the role of the state is crucial in supporting and enforcing the ideology. In other words, rather than giving benediction to the monopoly created naturally out of the needs of society, as Parson would have it, the state works with the profession in creating the monopoly by adopting and enforcing the profession's ideology.

Unlike Berlant and Freidson who concentrate on medicine, Magali Sarfatti Larson analyzes professionalization as a general phenomenon. She draws a great deal on Freidson's insights, particularly his analysis of how a profession produces an ideology. However, Larson approaches the problem from the standpoint of the development of capitalism and the market system. Thus she sees professionalization "as a process by which producers of a special service sought to constitute and control a market for their expertise." [25] The result is a new kind of structural inequality in society and expertise becomes (along with property) a way of defining class. Special technical knowledge becomes a new "scarce resource." [26] Larson also has a new view of the origins of professional ideology which she sees as arising from a need to keep the expertise surrounded with barriers so that it remains scarce.

According to Larson, the model or image of a profession was formed before it became commonplace in all of society, but the development of monopoly capitalism provided the means by which the ideology of professionalization could become extended to all sectors of the population. For Larson, the nature of the profession is determined by how its ideology is defined. The expertise is defined by the elites and gradually extended down to the lower ranks. Those at the bottom of the profession tend to adopt the ideas of the elites because such adoption secures their economic interest. Thus by adopting a professional definition of expertise they are also at the same time buying economic security.

Larson sees modern scientific and technological developments as playing the role of affirmation. In monopoly capitalism science and technology have promoted growth to a level where it is at least felt in terms of a rise in the average standard of living. Thus a wider sector of the population feels the effects of science and technology and has come to see it as "a permanent and indisputable system of cognitive and ideological validation." [27]

For Larson, as for Freidson, the role of the state is crucial. In marked contradiction to Parson, Freidson and Larson see no inherent contradiction between state intervention and professional development. Larson points out that professions are not inherently anti-bureaucratic. She emphasizes that the traditional view of the relationship between the professions and bureaucracy derives from the Weberian model of bureaucracy as rational and legal. In this traditional view, bureaucracy is seen as inherently antithetical to the supposedly autonomous, self-regulating professions. However, as Larson points out, in practice bureaucracy and the professions have come to depend upon one another and tend to seek an equilibrium in their relationship. Modern techno-bureaucracy, like the professions, relies on expertise as a supporting ideology. Thus the professions and bureaucracy reinforce each other. Professions provides the authority of the defined expertise, and the bureaucracy supplies regulations, laws, and support mechanisms to assure the professional monopoly.

This study constitutes an excellent test case for the theories of Parson, Berlant, Freidson and Larson. While agreeing with Freidson that ideology is important in the professionalization process, I do not see the bacteriological revolution as playing the role he ascribes to it in the process of the professionalization of French physicians. While it is certainly true that the bacteriological revolution helped to change the attitude of the state and the public toward the medical profession, it does not seem to have been terribly important, internally, to professional ideology. The professional ideology was defined on much less explicit grounds. Rather than a coherent theory of practice, French physicians in this period developed an image of their social role which was the rallying point for broader professionalization. According to this image, the physician perfomed a critical social service for which he should receive respect, adequate financial compensation, and special status from the state. The image stressed individuality in practice, and encouraged the physician to rely on his personal judgment. Finally, the image pictured medical care as a personal, private encounter between doctor and client, or doctor and family, which should be compensated for directly by the parties concerned on a fee for service basis.

This study supports Larson's contention that professional concepts were formed early in the development of market capitalism by the profession's elite, and were then extended to the lower orders of the profession during a later phase of economic development which included the growth of monopolies. The timing of these developments in France would tend to support Larson's model, although it is not at all clear that the French economy was truly entering into a phase of monopoly capitalism in the late nineteenth century. It must also be stressed that the general practitioners who achieved their desired professional status in the late nineteenth century did not adopt a model of the profession identical to that created about one hundred years earlier by the profession's elite. It was axiomatic to their movement that certain changes must be made in France's medical system in order for the private practitioners to achieve their own version of professionalism.

As Berlant and Freidson have noted, the attitude of the profession toward the health reforms of the bacteriological revolution was ambiguous. While not at all reluctant to identify with the scientific advancements made by Pasteur, Lister and Koch, and with the work of active public health reformers such as Paul Brouardel and A.J. Martin, private practitioners nevertheless actively opposed many public health reforms. Certainly there is evidence to support Berlant and Freidson's contentions that this opposition was motivated by a conflicting vision of medical care, in other words, the physician's emphasis on treating the individual rather than society as a whole. Yet their opposition to public health did not mean that the private physicians completely rejected state intervention. In accordance with the insights of Freidson and Larson, the profession and the growing public assistance and public health bureaucracy sought to resolve their differences and establish an equilibrium. The lower orders of the medical profession had a model to follow in the elites of the profession who had achieved the successful coexistance of state intervention and private practice. The lower orders sought the same sort of harmony, but with less state intervention into doctor-patient relationships. They also sought state legislation to extend their monopoly over medical practice, to facilitate the collection of fees and to make it possible for private, licensed, medical practice to be established in parts of the nation which had previously been unable or unwilling to support it.

The average private practitioners had sought this sort of legislative support for several decades. [28] In the 1880's the relationship between the state and private practitioners changed dramatically, making possible the realization of these goals. The change in the state's attitude occurred out of the political and social issues which seemed critical for the preservation of the Third Republic. And it changed because private practitioners were able to organize their own political lobbying force, distinct from that of the elites, to guide the concerns of the government into the directions which private physicians thought the future of medical care should take. Jacques Donzelot has argued that the state of the Third Republic formed an alliance with private practitioners with the goal of transforming the family life of the lower classes in order to "moralize and normalize" it according to middle class norms. [29] As Donzelot describes, by the 1920s French doctors had established a firm role for themselves as expert witnesses in court cases and in the social service network, where they defined acceptable and unacceptable behavior in individuals and described proper family relations. Besides coming to dominate the interventionist-helping professions, doctors also affected the structures of the medical care delivery system itself.

Theodore Zeldin has pointed out that the social reforms of the 1890s have been largely ignored by historians. [30] The traditional view of the period is one of stalemate and stagnation. [31] However, between 1888 and 1902 the Third Republic legislatures passed numerous pieces of social reform legislation. Three of these laws effected the medical system and are the subjects of this study: the 1892 Law on the Practice of Medicine (Loi Chevandier), the Medical Assistance Law of 1893, and the 1902 Public Health Law. The reform period began with a burst of social legislation in the period 1892-1893 which dealt with working conditions among factory workers in general and limitation on work hours for women and children, as well as the medical issues of professional practice, medical assistance and public health. [32] The reform movement was also responsible for the Méline Tariff, the 1898 Law on mutual aid societies and the 1898 Law on employer responsibility for work accidents. Zeldin states that the reform movement of this period failed, but this is not altogether correct. It is true that no dramatic transformation of society took place, but as Zeldin himself notes, this was never the aim of most of the reformers involved. [33]

The goals of the reformers of the period must be understood by an examination of the ideology of solidarism. As J.E.S. Hayward has pointed out, solidarism made it possible for legislators and bureaucrats of diverse political viewpoints to unite to initiate social reform under the Third Republic. [34] Solidarism is principally known as the ideology of the radical party after about 1895; its primary exponent was the radical leader who became prime minister in that year, Léon Bourgeois. Bourgeois took a very active role in medical issues and was Minister of the Interior when the Medical Practice Law and the Medical Assistance Law were drawn up in that ministry. Bourgeois was also the co-founder of the Permanent Anti-Tuberculosis Committee. In spite of the crucial role of Bourgeois and other radicals, solidarist ideology and medical reform appealed to members of a wide political spectrum. Solidarist slogans were expressed by progressives like Raymond Poincaré, opportunists like Jules Siegfried, moderates like Jules Méline and independent socialists like Alexandre Millerand. Its diverse appeal can be explained by its diverse origins, which included the thought of Louis Blanc, Proudhon, and Joseph de Maistre. [35]

Solidarists were unified by the perception that in order to endure the Third Republic had to find a third way between socialism and laissez-faire capitalism. [36] The development of solidarist reform in 1888-1902 must be understood in light of two major threats facing the ruling middle class elite: populationism and socialism. These two problems were intrinsically linked in the minds of the ruling elite and their efforts to counteract them inspired the medical reform legislation. Republicans were shaken by the strikes and Boulangist agitation of the period 1888-1893, and by the success of the socialists in the municipal elections of 1892 and in the legislative elections of 1893. These developments forced a general recognition of the need for social reform. Further, the distress of the rural population due to the agricultural crises of the period help to diminish faith in economic liberalism. At the same time, the Ralliement threatened to create a conservative ideology of reform which would capitalize on the unrest of the lower classes. The solidarist solution was to develop an ideology of reform that was "opposed equally to liberal economism, Marxist collectivism, Catholic corporatism and anarchist syndicalism." [37] The aim of solidarism was to achieve, in the words of Léon Bourgeois, "social peace through justice." [38]

Solidarist reform was also inspired by the scientific developments of the late ninteteenth century which seemed to hold out renewed hope for social progress. Solidarism consciously rejected Spencer's social Darwinism and sought active solutions for what Durkheim called cultural anomie brought about by the loss of traditional social structures based upon family and church. Solidarism stressed the view that the individual and society were organically linked by obligatory duties toward one another. Rather than independence, the goal of the government was to acknowledge the interdependence of all of its citizens and to lead, or even force, its citizens to carry out their obligations to one another. Thus state assistance or at least mutual cooperation should replace voluntary charity in aiding the unfortunate.

At bottom, the goals of solidarism were profoundly conservative in that they intended to make no fundamental change in either the economic or social systems. Solidarism was essentially a program to make the peasants and working class more like the bourgeoisie. As Jean Jaurès noted in his comments on the solidarist backed Méline Tariff, the reforms of the 1890s amounted to a slightly different rendition of Guizot's solution for the distress of the lower classes, "Enrichissez-vous." [39] The popular philosopher, Izoulet, explained that the goal of solidarist was to "prevent the crowd from overthrowing the elite, while yet admitting the crowd 'loyally and cordially into the state.'" [40] Solidarists were by no means seeking to equalize all members of society, and they had no desire to abolish private property or to attack capitalism. Rather they sought to improve the chances of working class families for a better life within the capitalist system by providing eduction, minimum wages, regulation of working hours, and limitations on the work of women and children. They also sought certain guarantees against the worst disasters which formerly devastated French families of the lower orders: illness, unemployment, work accidents, and old age. [41]

Populationist anxiety was an equally important element of solidarist reforms. By 1888, French elites had worked themselves into a frenzied fear that the end of French society was in sight because of the low reproductive rates of the population. In reality the population was never in real danger of disappearing and was actually continuing to grow in the late nineteenth century (5.4% between 1881 and 1911). [42] The anxieties over population resulted from the comparison of France, Germany and Britain for it was clear that the French were reproducing themselves at nowhere near the rate of their neighbors.

An important aspect of French populationism was concern over specific internal trends. By the 1890s it was apparent that the urban population was growing at the expense of the rural. [43] To the Republican elites this meant that the source of its troubles, the working class, was increasing in numbers, while the source of much of its support, the peasantry, was diminishing. [44] This could only mean the growth of socialism at the expense of radicals, progressives, and moderates. Thus the population question and the social question were inherently linked. There was a direct connection between such seemingly diverse projects as the Méline Tariff of 1892 and the Medical Assistance Law of 1893: both were part of solidarist efforts to preserve the peasantry.

There were of course marked differences among the various proponents of solidarist principles. Left-wing radicals, radical-socialists, and independent socialists advocated serious state interventionism supported by a progressive income tax. Most radicals also desired an income tax but supported a more limited reform program which provided for some state intervention but which put more faith in social mutualism. Mutualism amounted to a sort of corporatism where employers, with some state encouragement, would help workers create insurance societies and pension programs. [45] Progressives and moderates generally backed radical-solidarist reforms but balked on the income tax, successfully blocking it. Nevertheless, much of the solidarist program was successfully enacted. Populationist concerns were used to push through the Medical Assistance Law of 1893, a law which was recognized at the time as a monument to solidarist ideology. These solidarist notions also entered into the arguments in favor of the 1892 Law on the Practice of Medicine as well as the 1902 Public Health Law. These medical reforms were issues which could unify radicals, moderates, progressives and even some socialists.

Solidarism and its political and populationist antecedents explain the intense interest of the French state, in the period 1888-1902, in the general issue of medical reform. The nature of that medical reform was determined by private practitioners themselves, acting through a professional Union movement which developed close ties and great influence with the governments of the Third Republic.

Although they did not hesitate to use solidarist and populationist arguments in favor of the reforms they desired, private medical practitioners had a very negative view of state interventionism and mutualism. The issue of state activism was one which separated the mass of general practitioners from the medical elites. The elites had benefited from the status offered by state positions and had promoted the state's role in medicine. But in the opinion of general practitioners, medical bureaucracy needed to be greatly modified. Rather than aspiring to government positions, most physicians wanted to see the practice of medicine separated from the status of *fonctionnaire*. Therefore, the suddenly renewed interest which the state took in medical matters in the late 1880s was both a boon and a threat to practitioners in the physicians' Union movement. The Union's goal was to harness state concern to their professional interest while raising barriers to state control over the medical system. They demanded state action which would protect and extend private practice while actively opposing the creation of a central bureaucracy to oversee public health and medical assistance, and working to reduce the role of hospitals and dispensaries in medical care. Thus the success of private practitioners in these areas meant the spread of liberal, private, market medicine at the expense of state-sponsored care and private pre-paid care.

As Jacques Léonard and others have pointed out, the Third Republic saw the rise of a large number of individual doctors to political prominence, a position they had not enjoyed in great numbers under the July Monarchy or Second Empire. [46] Certainly this was of great benefit to physicians in expanding professionalization. However, it was not the only factor or even the crucial factor. As subsequent chapters will show, although certain physician-deputies worked very hard to promote the professional goals of physicians, the mass of doctors found they could not rely on all of their colleagues in the legislature. Locally, activist doctors found they could not rely on the practitioner-representatives to the departmental councils either. Many of the politician-doctors came from the very medical elite which had profited from the tradition of state and medical elite alliance. Often these doctors had no understanding or sympathy for the opposition of the mass of practitioners to increased state involvement in medical practice.

The keys to the promotion of the professional interests of doctors lay in two other developments: the formation of the physicians' Union movement and the Union's effective promotion of its goals in the public assistance bureaucracy. As R. D. Anderson notes, the policy-making activities of civil servants is a neglected aspect of the history the Third Republic. [47] Although the legislature had numerous permanent and *ad hoc* committees which drafted legislation, the medical legislation of this period was drawn up largely in the public health and public assistance bureaucracies. This study, then, focuses on the development of the physicians' syndicats and Union and their effect on the programs of these bureaucracies. The study will show that the private practitioners' Union was organized with an awareness that the political and social atmosphere of the Third Republic in the era of the 1880 and 1890s was highly favorable to new medical legislation and programs and, if managed correctly, these could be guided to promote private practice and stave off the threat of an expansion of state medicine. This organization was as decisive in determining the future of French medicine as the physicians organizing it intended. The Union was responsible for the enactment of two pieces of medical legislation: the 1892 Medical Practice Law (Loi Chevandier) and the 1893 Medical Assistance Law. The Union was also critically influential in the formulation of a third Law, the 1902 Public Health Law. This study will focus on the Union's role in these three pieces of medical legislation and its effect on other public

health programs. It will focus also on the interplay of professional concerns and political issues which together describe the medical politics of
the era.

NOTES TO THE INTRODUCTION

1. Eugen Weber, *Peasants Into Frenchmen, The Modernization of Rural France, 1870-1914,* 1976. Standard works referred to include: Francois Goguel, *La politique des partis sous la IIIe République,* 1956; Jacques Chastenet, *Histoire de la Troisième République,* 1974; Robert David Anderson, *France, 1870-1914; Politics and Society,* 1977; Jean-Pierre Azéma and Michel Winock, *La IIIe République, Naissance et Mort,* 1970; Denis William Brogan, *The Development of Modern France,* V. I, 1974; Guy Chapman, *The Third Republic of France, The First Phase 1871-1894;* Jean Mayeur, *Débats de la Troisième République,* 1871-1898, 1973; David Thomson, *Democracy in France;* Madelaine Reberioux, *La République Radicale?, 1898-1914,* 1975; Theodore Zeldin, *France 1848-1945,* V. 1, 1973. In the last mentioned work, Zeldin discusses physicians at length but leaves out the political and medical impact of their increasing political influence.

2. The concept of hybridization is drawn from Gilles Deleuze, foreward to Jacques Donzelot, *The Policing of Families,* 1979.

3. Talcott Parsons, "Social change and medical organization in the United States," *The Annals of the American Academy of Political and Social Science,* V. 346, (March 1963), pp 21-33; "The Professions and

Social Structure" in *Essays in Sociological Theory,* 1954; Eliot Freidson, *Profession of Medicine, A Study of Applied Knowledge,* 1970;
Jacques Léonard, *La France médicale au XIX siècle.*

4. The Royal Society of Medicine, founded by the Turgot Ministry in
1774 was "discovered" by historian Jean Meyer in 1966 and became the
stimulus to an exciting burst of research into the social history of medicine in France. The archives of the Royal Society have provided
numerous insights into the medical concerns and ideology of the late
eighteenth century. The Royal Society was founded in an effort to
escape from the retrograde constraints of the Faculty of Medicine which
had become a barrier to the development the science of medicine in
France. Gelfand argues that the Royal Society can be seen therefore as
the direct precursor of the breakthroughs in medical thought achieved
by the clinical school of Paris after the Revolution: Toby Gelfand, *Professionalizing Modern Medicine, Paris Surgeons and Medical Science
and Institutions in the 18th Century,* 1980. Jean-Pierre Peter, however,
has pointed out that in its ideology the Royal Society never went
beyond traditional climatological notions of disease. Peter sees its
major significance in its unprecedent information gathering efforts
which successfully amassed a tremendous archive of information about
the health of the French people. Jean-Pierre Peter, "Une enquête de la
Société Royale de Médecine (1774-1794): Malades et maladies à la fin
du XVIII siècle," *Annales, Economies, Sociétés et Civilisations,*
(hereinafter, AESC), (July-Aug. 1967). Peter has also used the Royal
Society archives to discuss the issue of the history of medical diagnostic

language: Peter, "Le Mots et les Objets de la maladie," *Revue His-torique* N. 499, (July-Sept., 1977), p 381. The efforts of the oyal Society demonstrate the interest the French state took in pubic health at this time, unprecedented among the states of Europe. The Royal Society recognized the issue of work related diseased and addressed the It sponsored efforts to promote breast feeding, better enfant care and the licensing of midwives: Arlette Farge, "Les Artisans malades de leur travail," *AESC,* V. 32, N. 5 (Sept.-Oct. 1977); Marie France Morel, "Ville et Compagne dans le discours médical sur la petite enfance du XVIII siècle," *AESC,* V. 32, N. 5, (Sept-Oct. 1977); Actually, as Morel demonstrates, the efforts of the French state to address the issue of enfant mortality go back to at least 1762 when in the aftermath of the publication of *Emile,* France was flooded with literature on child health and child rearing. Jacques Gélis has shown that there was an active movement toward reform of childbirth practices beginning around 1728 with a series of inquiries initiated by the crown into midwivery: Jacques Gélis, "Sages-femmes et accoucheurs," *AESC,* V. 32, N. 5, (Sept.-Oct. 1977).

5. Toby Gelfand, *Ibid.;* David M. Vess, *Medical Revolution in France 1789-1796,* 1975; see also Jean-Pierre Peter, "Le Grand Rêve de l'ordre médical en 1770 et aujourd'hui," *Autrement,* N. 4, (1975/76), pp 183-192.

6. Gelfand, *Ibid.*

7. Gelfand, *Ibid.* In his seminal work, *The Birth of the Clinic,* 1973, Foucault argued that a dramatic transformation of medical thought

occurred among the members of the clinical school of medicine at the Paris hospitals in the early nineteenth century, under the leadership of Pinel and Bichat. This transformation had far reaching medical and political consequences, but it was primarily a transformation in the epistomology of disease concepts. It established the notion of disease as a social concept, and the body as its physicial location and place of study. However, there was still no unified theory of the causation of disease. As Léonard and Erwin Ackerknecht have both pointed out, Pinel and Bichat were by no means universally approved of among elite doctors of the nineteenth century who throughout the century maintained a proclivity for exploring diverse and conflicting theories of disease. Léonard, *La France médicale,* p 120; Erwin Ackerknecht, *Medicine at the Paris Hospital, 1794-1848* (1967). Vess and Gelfand have added another dimension to this period by discussing medical practice and professional development. However, Vess ignores the Royal Society of Medicine altogether. His thesis that a revolution in medical ideology originated on the battlefield simply ignores too many other factors. Gelfand's work is more insightful. He is certainly justified in stressing the importance of the synthesis between surgery and medicine which took place at this time. However, his thesis that a uniform medical ideology emerged during this time period remains problematic. Gelfand is more convincing when he argues that a concept of professionalization developed during the late 18th century.

8. Jacques Léonard, *Les Médecins de l'Quest au XIX siècle,* Thèse de doctorate d'Etat (University of Paris, 1975); also *La France Médicale*

au XIX Siècle (1978); Léonard, R. Darquenne and L. Bergeron, "Médecins et Notables sous le Consultat et l'Empire," *AESC,* (Sept.-Oct. 1977); J.P. Goubert, "The Extent of Medical Practice in France Around 1780," *Journal of Social History,* (Summer 1977); "L'Art de Guerir. Médecine savante et médecine populaire dans la France de 1790," *AESC* (Sept.-Oct. 1977); Matthew Ramsey, "Medical Power and Popular Medicine; Illegal healers in 19th Century France," *Journal of Social History* (Summer 1977); George Weisz, "The Politics of Medical Professionalization in France 1845-1848," *Journal of Social History* (Fall 1978); it is important to note that most of the work which has contributed to establising a picture of the social and economic status of the mass of medical practitioners, that is, the work of Léonard and Goubert, focuses only on French doctors in the Brittany and part of Normandy.

9. Eugen Weber, *Peasants into Frenchmen,* 1976; Martine Segalen, *Marie et femme dans la société paysanne,* 1980; Georges Dupeux, *French Society 1789-1907,* 1976.

10. Harvey Mitchell, "Rationality and control in French Eighteenth Century Medical Views of the Peasantry," *Comparative Studies in Society and History* (Jan, 1979), p 82.

11. See Chapter I below. The Royal Society of Medicine corresponded with a large number of rural practitioners, however, their main concern was gathering information about the health of the French people. The Society was not interested in transforming the status of the private practitioners.

12. David Higgs, "Le Dépôt de Mendacité de Toulouse, (1811-1818), *Annales du Midi,* V. 86, N. 119, (Oct.-Dec. 1974), p 403; Jean-Pierre Goubert, *Malades et Médecins en Bretagne, 1770-1790* 1974; "Eaux publique et démographie historique dans la France urbaine du XIX siècle. Le cas de Rennes," *Démographie historique* (1975); Pierre Lunel, "Pouvoir royal et Santé publique à la veille de la révolution. L'exemple du Rousillon," *Annales du Midi* V. 86, N. 119, (Oct.-Nov. 1974); T. Adams, "Moeurs et hygiène publique à Toulouse au début de XX siècle,: *Annales de Démographie Historique,* (1975) pp 131-137; Olivier Faure, "Physicians in Lyon during the Nineteenth Century, An Extraordinary Social Success," *Journal of Social History,* V. 10, N. 3, (summer 1977); Alan Forrest, "Le Révolution et les hopitaux dans le département de la Gironde," *Annales du Midi* V. 86, N. 119, (Oct.-Dec. 1974).

13. Léonard, *La France médicale.*

14. George Weisz, *Ibid.*

15. Ramsey, *Ibid.,* Weisz, *Ibid.*

16. Rene Dubois, *The Mirage of Health: Utopian Progress and Biological Change,* 1959; Ivan Illich, *Medical Nemesis, The Expropriation of Health,* 1976; Thomas McKeown, *The Modern Rise of Population,* 1976; McKeown and R.G. Record, "Reasons for the Decline of Mortality in England and Wales During the Nineteenth Century," *Population Studies,* XVI (1962-63), p 24; McKeown and R.G. Brown, "Medical Evidence Related to English Population Changes in the Eighteenth Century," *Population Studies,* IX, (1955-56); McKeown and Gordon

McLachlan, eds, *Medical History and Medical Care: A Symposium of Perspectives,* 1971; for a bibliographical essay on the literature on the subject of medical effectiveness see: John Powles, "On the Limitations of Modern Medicine," in *Science, Medicine and Man* 1973.

17. Thomas McKeown, "A Sociological Approach to the History of Medicine," in McKeown and McLachlan, *Ibid.*

18. Jacques Léonard, *La France médicale au XIX sìecle,* (1978) p 225; *Les Médecins du l'Quest au XIX sìecle,* V. IV, p 28. Although the hygiene literature no doubt had some effect on the health practices of the middle classes it is difficult to believe that such books made much impact on the lower classes. More important in changing the health habits of workers and peasants was the hygiene lessons which were increasingly given in public schools during the Third Republic. Workers were no doubt also affected by the campaigns of the anti-alcohol leagues. These leagues were were made up to a significant extent by elite physicians.

19. McKeown, Ibid, p 6.

20. Jeffrey Berlant, *Profession and Monopoly, A Study of Medicine in the United States and Great Britain,* 1975; Eliot Freidson, *Profession of Medicine, A Study of the Sociology of Applied Knowledge,* 1970; Magali Sarfatti Larson, *The Rise of Professionalism,* 1977. Berlant's work is a historical sociology of the profession of medicine in the United States and Great Britain. Freidson's works is a very insightful analysis of the way physicians in the United States today relate to each other, their patients, society and the state. Larsons' work, also critically important,

is a historically informed interpretation of the general phenomenon of professions in the modern industrialized west. A very useful historical analysis and critique of Talcott Parsons and structural functionalism can be found in: Alvin Gouldner, *The Coming Crisis in American Sociology* 1970. Gouldner provides a history of the discipline of sociology and describes the social and political influences that shaped the American academic sociology.

21. Freidson, *Ibid*, p 170, Freidson notes that the dominant style of medical training, the clinical method, emphasizes direct experience over the acquisition of a body of "book learned" theory and principles. Therefore the individual practitioner is encouraged to trust his own experiences and the conclusions he derives from them over general principles or scientific developments.

22. Christopher Lasch, *Haven in a Heartless World, The Family Beseiged,* 1977; Jacques Donzelot, *The Policing of Families,* foreward by Gillis Deleuze, trans: Robert Hurley, 1979 *(La Police des Familles,* 1977).

23. Freidson, *Ibid.* p 5.

24. Freidson, *Ibid.* p 15.

25. Larson, *Ibid.* p xvi.

26. *Ibid.* p xvii.

27. Larson, *Ibid,* p 200.

28. Battling with the state for power over the medical realm was a well established issue for the mass of French doctors. General works on this

issue include: T. Adams, "Moeurs et hygiène publique au XVIII siècle. Quelques aspects de dépôts de mendacité," *Annales de Démographie hisorique,* 1975, pp 93-105; A. Armengaud, "Avant Propos: Misère, maladies et assistance," *Annales de Midi,* T. 86; N. 119; (Oct-Dec. 1974); "Quelques Aspects de l'hygiène publique de Toulouse au début de XX siècle," *Annales de Démographie historique* (1975), pp 131-137; J.N. Biraben, "La Diffusion de la Vaccinations en France au XIX siècle," *Annales de Bretagne,* T. 86, N. 2, (June 79); Alain Corbin, "Le Péril vénérien au début du siècle: prophylaxie sanitaire et prophylaxie morale," *Récherches, l'Haleine des Faubourgs* N. 29, (Dec 1977); J.P. Desaive, et. al., *Médecins, climat, et épidémies à la fin du XVIII siècle,* 1972; Arlette Farge, "Les Artisans malades de leur Travail," *AESC,* 1977, N. 5, (Sept-Oct.); Faure, *Ibid;* Forrest, *Ibid;* Goubert, *Ibid.;* Higgs, *Ibid;* Anne Fowler La Berge, "The French Public Health Movement," *Proceedings of the Annual Meeting of the Western Society for French* History, N. 3, (1975), pp 337-353; Léonard, Ibid; Lunel, *Ibid;* Panzac, *Ibid;* Peter, *Ibid;* George Sussman, "From Yellow Fever to Cholera, A Study of French Government Policy, Medical Professionalism, and Popular Movements in the Epidemic Crisis of the Restoration and the July Monarchy," (unpublished Ph.D. dissertation, Yale University, 1971); also "Enlightened Health Reform, Professional Medicine and Traditional Society: The Cantonal Physicians of the Bas-Rhin, 1810-1870" *Bulletin of the History of Medicine,* Vol. 51, N. 4, (1977), p 565; R. Heller, "Officiers de santé, the Second-class Doctors of Nineteenth Century France," *Medical History,* V. 1, N. 22, (Jan 1978) pp 25-43; J.P. Peter, "Le Grand Rêve de L'Ordre médical en 1770 et aujourd'hui," *Autrement*, N. 4, 1975/76, pp 183-192; Weisz, *Ibid*. After the 1845 medical congress a new law on the practice of medicine, abolishing the second order of practitioners, was introduced by Minister of Education Salvandy. This bill made it through the *Chambre des Pares* and was awaiting action in the Chamber of Deputies when the revolution of 1848 broke out. See Ramsey, *Ibid*.

29. Donzelot, *Ibid.*, p 84. Since this manuscript was first written, Robert Nye has added an important new analysis of the issue of medicine and social reform in the Third Republic, see: Robert Nye, *Crime, Madness and Politics in Modern France: The Medical Concept of National Decline,* Princeton University Press: 1984.

30. Zeldin, *Ibid,* p 641.

31. Stanley Hoffman, *In Search of France;* Francois Goguel, *La Politique des Parties sous la IIIe république,* p 17; "Six Authors in Search of a National Character," *In Search of France,* Stanley Hoffman, et.at. eds. p 395; David Thompson, *Democracy in France.*

32. Law of November 2, 1892 on working hours for women and children, which also set a minimum age of 13 for child workers; Law of June 12, 1893 which regulated the cleanlines and safety of factories. Also in 1893 the Chamber of Deputies passed a law on public health which was subsequently refused by the Senate because it went too far in giving the public health bureaucracy control over the declaration of dangerous housing.

33. Zeldin, *Ibid.*

34. J.E.S. Hayward, "Solidarity: The Social History of an Idea in Nineteenth Century France," *International Review of Social History,* Vol. IV, (1959) Part 1, p 281.

35. Hayward, *Ibid.,* p 261-284.

36. Henri Hatzfeld, *Du Paupérisme a la sécurité sociale, Essai sur les origines de la sécurité sociale, 1850-1940;* Robert David Anderson, *France, 1870-1914: Politics and Society,* 1977, pp 95-98; Theodore Zeldin, *France 1848-1945, V. 1, Ambition, Love and Politics* pp 641-660; J.E.S. Hayward, "The Official Philosophy of the French Third Republic: Léon Bourgeois and Solidarism," *International Review of Social History,* V. 6 (1961), pp 19-48; "Solidarity: The Social History of an Idea in Nineteenth Century France," *International Review of Social History,* V. IV, Part 2, (1959), pp 261-84.

37. J.E.S. Hayward, "The Official Philosophy of the French Third Republic: Léon Bourgeois and Solidarism," *Ibid,* p 19.

38. *Ibid.,* p 20.

39. Goldberg, *The Life of Jean Jaurès,* pp 181-82.

40. Zeldin, *Ibid,* p 659.

41. Hayward, *Ibid.,* p 34. As Hayward points out, most of these principles were embodied in the radical party electoral program of 1891 which brought them modest success in the 1893 elections.

42. A.S. (1930), pp 12.

43. This development was the result of industrial expansion but more importantly it was the result of the prolonged agricultural crisis of the 1880s and 1890s: Gordon Wright, *Rural Revolution in France.*

44. Jules Ferry noted in 1885: "The Republic will be the Republic of the Peasants or it will be nothing," R.D. Anderson, *Ibid,* p 94.

45. Méline was the best example of a profoundly conservative republican who yet, while, Prime Minister promoted the work Accident Law of 1898 because he saw it as a way of promoting insurance societies.

46. Léonard, Roger Darquenne and Jacques Bergeron, "Médecins et Notables sous le consultat et l'Empire, *AESC,* V. 32, N. 5, (Sept-Oct, 1977), pp 858-865.

47. R.D. Anderson, *Ibid,* p 81.

CHAPTER I
FRENCH DOCTORS 1888-1902:
A PROFESSION IN CRISIS

At the turn of the century French doctors enjoyed unprecedented social influence and political success, yet paradoxically, they felt threatened and oppressed. At the same time that doctors were basking in the reflected glory of Louis Pasteur, the pages of the professional medical press were full of lamentations about the crisis faced by private practitioners. [1] According to the doctors, their crisis was characterized by loss of status, difficulties in finding clients and making a living, and unwanted changes in traditional medical practices. Some of the doctors' complaints revolved around problems which were decades old: over-crowding in the profession, unregulated competition of legal and illegal practitioners, and inadequate fees. However, developments in this period brought new threats to the profession. Concern over depopulation and the implications of the bacteriological revolution sparked a movement to create a centralized public health bureaucracy and an accompanying corps of *médecins-fonctionnaires*. Medical advances had resulted in the increased use of hospitals, and a plethora of new public services including disinfection, dispensaries, and sanatoriums. To private practitioners it seemed that these changes would hurt the profession by usurping clienteles and increasing the state's role in medical care. In the face of these threats they created a national professional Union movement which turned the crisis into triumph. Through this movement doctors ovecame their old problems and greatly reduced the perceived threats of the nascent public health bureaucracy. In doing so private practitioners of the Union movement profoundly affected the development of modern medical care in France. Some traditional attributes of the official medical care system were diminished by their movement: the hierarchy within the profession, and the established role of state bureaucracies. Private practitioners also achieved a true monopoly over medical care by moving licensed practice into the poorer echelons of society. This was accomplished through both the 1892 Medical Practice Law and the 1893 Medical Assistance Law. Before discussing these two acts in more detail, this chapter will describe the organization of the Union movement, and the way in which it voiced the perceived crisis within the profession and laid out a plan for its cure.

The crisis perceived by private practitioners of the 1880s and 1890s was very similar in its themes to complaints made two generations earlier. In 1845, private practitioners held a medical congress to discuss grievances and write new regulations on medical practice. The doctors wanted to expand their monopoly over medical pracice which meant the elimination of illegal practitioners, the abolition of the second order of doctors, the *officiers de santé,* and greater restrictions on the practice of other licensed practitioners such as midwives, pharmacists and dentists. In the 1880s and 1890s, physicians were still pursuing the same goals; however, their program to achieve these goals had changed dramatically. In 1845, unsuccessfully as it turned out, doctors counted on convincing the Ministry of Education to support their program and seek legislation in their favor. [2] In the Third Republic, private physicians created their own political power base to lobby directly to the legislature, bureaucracy and courts.

In 1845 many doctors still counted on an increase in state sponsored jobs for doctors to solve the problem of an overcrowded profession. Thus the 1845 movement has been described as "neo-corporatist" rather than "professional-protectionist." [3] The professional movement of the Third Republic, however, was clearly professional-protectionist. It aimed at promoting the practice of medicine as a liberal profession, based upon a private, contractual relationships between doctor and clients where the doctor would be paid directly for services rendered. By this time, most private practitioners were strongly opposed to any collective form of medical care, whether it be state programs or pre-paid private care systems. But these same doctors actively sought state intervention in the form of legislative and bureaucratic support for private medicine.

Another difference between the 1845 movement and the movement of 1888-1902 was that the later movement emanated to a far greater extent from private practitioners. These practitioners saw their interests as quite distinct from the interests of the profession's elite consisting of physicians connected to the Faculties of Medicine, Academy of Medicine, and government bureaucracies. Private practitioners believed that the medical elites, whose status was the result of their connections with the state, would benefit from the continued bureaucratization of medical care. The less favored members of the profession who were entirely dependent on private practice for their income had come to believe that their best interest lay in reducing the role of the state in medical care. They realized that in order to do so they must reject, to a certain extent, the traditional leaders of the profession and find new leadership from among themselves.

The physicians' Union movement originated in the Paris basin and spread quickly throughout the country. The movement began in 1879 with the founding the journal *Le Concours médical* by Dr. Auguste Cézilly (1833-1903). Cézilly had an enormous impact on medical developments in this period. Through *Le Concours* he guided the professional debates of the period, promoted the medical syndicat movement and had a great influence on the medical legislation of the period. His biography illustrates the occupational experiences which typified the practitioners of the syndicat movement and separated them from the medical elites.

Cézilly came from the remote Basses-Alpes. Through his career as a navy surgeon and service in the Crimean War, he moved from the provinces toward Paris. [4] In 1858 Cézilly began the private practice of medicine in Chantilly, "leading the rude existence of the doctor of a small country village." [5] Cézilly took an active part in the defense of France in 1870 and was imprisoned by the Prussians. An ardent Republican, he was elected village mayor in 1876. Because of his growing concern over the situation of the rural private practitioners, Cézilly abandoned regular politics in 1879 in favor of medical politics. The founding of *Le Concours médical* in that year amounted to a revolution in medical journalism. Unlike the established and prestigious medical press of Paris and Bordeaux, Cézilly's journal was aimed mainly at professional issues with science as secondary matter. The writers of *Le Concours* dealt with economic and social issues never touched by the established medical press represented by the *Gazette des Hôpitaux,* the *Gazette médicale de Paris,* and the *Gazette Hebdomandaire des Sciences médicale de Bordeaux.*

Cézilly later became one of the founders of the Association de la Presse médicale française, but was never really accepted as an equal by the Paris medical press establishment. His death in 1902, although mourned at length by the members of *Le Concours* and the Union movement, went virtually unremarked by the rest of the medical press. This same press, however, printed lengthy eulogies upon the death of Dr. Henri Roger, the president of the older and more established professional organization, the A.G.M.F. (Association générale des Médecins français). [6] Dr. J. Noir's commentary on this snub by the established press illustrates the hostility felt by private practitioners toward the profession's elite:

"It is simply the proof of a fact that we have maintained thousands of times; this indifference from the great majority of the organs of the medical press is a witness to their indifference to professional interests and private practitioners. They fill their columns with exposés of pseudo-scientific work, phony titles which are aimed at giving such an such official personage the appearance of a scientific genius. They relate with banal praise the careers of the good men of the court who, once they finish the intrigues of their life, justifiably fall into eternal oblivion, but they do not find it worthy to include in their gallery an independent man of strong intelligence and energetic character who came to wake an entire profession from a dangerous sleep and create thousands of useful projects for a crowd of miserable private practitioners and inspire them with feelings of dignity and a realization of the collective force with which they could impose this respect everywhere." [7]

According to Cézilly, the idea for *Le Concours* originated with a group of doctors from Paris and nearby departments whom he gathered together in 1877 to discuss the problems of the profession. They decided to form a national professional organization different from both the French A.G.M.F. and the British Medical Association. Cézilly and his group felt that both of these models had serious faults. The A.G.M.F. mainly functioned as an insurance society for doctors, providing pensions and survivor's benefits, while the British Medical Association was aimed solely at pursuing professional interests. Cézilly and his group decided to found a society which combined these two functions. The result was the *Société civile du Concours médical,* founded in 1880 as an organization which would address professional and medical-political issues and would also provide economic aid and protection.

Cézilly and the society began a pension plan and other protective associations, which put *Le Concours* in clear competition with the A.G.M.F. [8]

Cézilly's success was impressive. He claimed to have received over one thousand subscriptions to the first issue of *Le Concours* in 1879, and by 1888 there were 3,455 practitioners receiving weekly issues. [9] The leadership of the society and the letters written to he journal support Cézilly's claim that the journal and society represented the views of private practitioners from all over the nation. Prominent leaders of the society in the 1890s were Drs. Gassot of Loiret, Porsons of Nantes (Loire-Inférieure), Mignen of Montaigu (Vendée), Bibard of Pointoise (Seine-et-Oise), Maurat of Chantilly (Oise), Fourmestreaux and Jeanne of Meulan (Seine-et-Oise), Grellety of Allier, Lasalle of Lormont (Gironde), and Lecuyer of Saint-Jean-d'Angely (Aisne). [10] In 1880 *Le Concours* started two projects, an inquiry into the "reasons for the impoverishment of private practitioners in France," and a project to revise the law of 1803 on the practice of medicine. [11] Members of the society felt that Cézilly had launched a virtual social revolution in the medical profession by promoting the professional interests of private pracitioners as distinct from those of the medical elites and the state. [12]

Very quickly Cézilly made some very important political connections among doctor-politicians: Deputy Antoine Daniel Chevandier who would sponsor the 1892 Law on the Practice of Medicine; Dr. Gibert, mayor and public health reformer of Havre who was a co-founder of the Union movement and a member of the National Public Assistance

Council; Dr. Lardier who was also a member of the National Public Assistance Council. Other collaborators included Senators Léon Labbé, Andre Victor Cornil, and Ludovic Trarieux; and the leader of the radical party, Waldeck-Rousseau. All of the former were members of Le Concours. In addition, Cézilly was an associate of two important health bureaucrats: the famous reformer, Theophile Roussel, and Henri Monod, long-time head of the public assistance bureaucracy. [13]

In 1881 the Le Concours group went a step further in its program to organize private practitioners and founded the Union des Syndicats médicaux de France. The idea of a syndicat movement among doctors reportedly began with Drs. Gibert and Margueritte of Le Havre who approached Cézilly in 1879 and received his eager cooperation. Cézilly and Le Concours quickly took over leadership of the movement. [14] Early Union leaders included Drs. Margueritte, Fourmestreaux, Barat-Dulaurier, and Jeanne, as well as Cézilly. [15] At this time unions were still illegal in France but at least two local physicians syndicats were founded before the Law of 1884 which legalized syndicalization. These were the Doctors' syndicat of Briode (Haute-Loire), founded in 1882 by Dr. Elie Noir and the syndicat of Montaigu (Vendée) founded by Dr. Mignen in 1884. [16] The Montaigu syndicat was the first to join the Union of syndicats. The Brioude syndicat was apparently short-lived; however, Dr. J. Noir, the son of its founder, went on to become a very active member of the Union of Syndicats and of Le Concours. Dr. J. Noir reported that he was brought up to worship Auguste Cézilly. [17]

The Union published its own bulletin separate from *Le Concours*. However, the two organizations, *Le Concours and the Union,* worked very closely together and in many ways were one and the same. Cézilly himself served as Vice-President of the Union. Union presidents of the 1880s and 1890s, Drs. Porson, Mignen, Barat-Dulaurier, Fourmestreaux, and Margueritte, also served on the board of *Le Concours*. In the early years, the governing boards of the two organizations were nearly identical. Other common members included Drs. H. Lecuyer of Beaurieux (Aisne), Maurat of Chantilly, Jeanne of Versaille, and Gibert of Havre who was honorary president of the Union. The dual organizations had useful aspects. In the early years before the Union movement gained momentum, *Le Concours* served as a sounding board for the concerns of private practitioners from all over the nation who were encouraged to write to the journal. Later, *Le Concours* served as an umbrella organization for several pension and insurance programs as well as some special organizations to pursue particular professional needs. For example, *Le Sou Médical* was organized to provide legal advice, lawyers, and pay the court expenses of doctors who became involved in any sort of court action involving the practice of medicine. A low yearly fee entitled practitioners to the services of the organization. Also, *Le Concours* organized the *Société pour les victimes du devoir médical,* a charitable organization to benefit the survivors of doctors who had died as a result of disease or injury contracted in the course of their medical practice. [18]

In the beginning of the movement, *Le Concours* led the way in political planning and lobbying. This was particularly true during the drafting and lobbying of 1892 Law on the Practice of Medicine. Eventually the Union took over this role, and *Le Concours* became more or less a forum for professional commentary, always in support of the Union, by an aging Cézilly and his chief collaborators. *Le Concours* also held an annual banquet meeting for members and supporters whose discussions serve as valuable indicators of professional concerns. The Union devoted itself more to organizing syndicats at the local level and lobbying in the department on medical issues thorugh this network of local syndicats.

In December 1884, the nascent syndicat movement received a serious blow when the Court at Caen, affirmed by the Cour de Cassation in June 1885, declared that doctors should not unionize. This decision received a strong and angry reaction from *Le Concours* and the Union, as well as from the established Paris medical press. Although the traditional medical journals had generally opposed the Union movement, they nevertheless resented the court's decision that physicians' unions posed some sort of threat to the nation. Dr. F. de Ranse, the editor of the prestigious *Gazette Médicale de Paris* was incensed that the courts would deem it more of a danger to the public interests when "learned and wise" men organized to protect their interests than when workers and commercial men did so. [19] The courts' decision made the syndicat doctors more determined and served to help publicize the movement. During the time that the courts were judging the issue of doctors' syndication, a new Law on the practice of medicine was being drawn up by a committee from the Chamber of Deputies under the leadership of Deputy-Dr. Chevandier. This law was presented to the Chamber in 1885 and contained an article legalizing unionization for doctors. This effectively put the issue of the unionization of doctors into legal suspension until such time as the bill would be considered.

It is difficult to determine accurately the size of the physicians' Union movement in the 1880s and 1890s. Information on the exact number of syndicat members is not readily available. It seems to have fluctuated greatly depending on the urgency of medical issues, and probably reached its height during the debates over medical assistance and insurance societies between 1895-1910. [20] The Belgian medical syndicat movement reported that the French Union included two hundred separate syndicats and 10,000 members by 1892. This figure is probably somewhat exaggerated since there were only about 14,000 doctors altogether in France at this time. [21]

Local syndicats belonging to the Union tended to be headquartered in small cities, suburbs and large areas of rural villages. For example, in Gironde the Union had syndicats in suburban Bordeaux, Reole, and the Medoc area (including Margaux and Saint-Laurent), but not in Bordeaux, whose very active syndicat was not part of the Union. [22] Seine-et-Oise was a stronghold of the Union movement with five syndicats belonging to the Union. [23] Seine-et-Oise also gave the movement several important leaders including Drs. Fourmestreaux and Jeanne. The syndicats belonging to the Union were geographically scattered, although there was a heavy concentration in the North and West. [24]

Many physicians' syndicats never joined the Union of Syndicats. In particular, the syndicats of major cities tended to keep independent from the Union. Many of these urban syndicats were involved in regional federations. The syndicat of Lyon sponsored its own Union of Syndicats in the region. [25] *La Fédération médicale* , headquartered in Toulouse, united ten syndicats in the area of the Garonne basin. [26] The very active Lille syndicat remained unaffiliated although two other syndicats in the same department belonged to the Union of Syndicats. The lack of complete national unity reflected some discord over the allocation of dues as well as the provincials' usual fear of being dominated by Paris. However in spite of a lack organizational unity, in practice the movement was very cohesive, rallying behind the promotion of a consistent legislative and professional agenda. [27]

The Union and the local syndicats often conflicted with the older established network of physicians' organizations affiliated with the A.G.M.F. The A.G.M.F., founded in 1858, was the oldest national physician's organization. By 1903 it had ninety-four local societies. [28] It was mainly concerned with providing insurance and pensions for doctors. Although the A.G.M.F. claimed in its founding documents that one of its goals was to combat illegal practice, private practitioners complained that it rarely did so. In addition to becoming involved in issues which the A.G.M.F. had generally avoided, *Le Concours* created rival pension and insurance plans. [29] By 1902, the pension plan of *Le Concours* was not as large as that of the A.G.M.F., having only a capital of 800,000 francs versus the four million francs of the A.G.M.F. However, it was steadily gaining members because of its intention to offer much larger pensions, 1200 francs a year after age sixty, versus the six to eight hundred offered by the A.G.M.F. plan. [30] In addition to pensions, the A.G.M.F. and *Le Concours* both had plans for illness insurance and survivors' benefits, but *Le Concours* made membership in thse plans available on a nation-wide basis for the first time.

Paris was the stronghold of the A.G.M.F., whose presidents were mainly drawn from the Conseil général des sociétés médicaux des arrondissements de Paris et du département de la Seine, the governing council which represented the medical societies of the Paris arrondissements and the Department of the Seine. The arrondissement and deparment medical societies were locals of the A.G.M.F. The *Le Concours* group struggled for three years to gain A.G.M.F. support for the syndicats, finally gaining its guarded official approval in 1892. [31] The president of the A.G.M.F., Dr. Odelon-Marc Lannelongue, still expressed strong misgivings about the syndicat movement because of its possibly negative impact on the public image of doctors. [32] Because of A.G.M.F. opposition, the syndicat movement did not attempt to move into Paris proper until 1891, over ten years after the founding of the first syndicats, in spite of the fact that *Le Concours* was actually head-quartered in Paris. Le Concours-Union personnel undoubtedly felt they had to gain some national momentum before taking on the Paris medical establishment. Finally, in 1891, Dr. Le Baron created the *Association syndicale professionelle des Médecins de la Seine* which was an instant success, gaining over two hundred members in its first six months of existence. This Paris syndicat caused a great debate over the need for a syndicat movement. [33] These controversies shed light upon the essential differences between the syndicat movment and the medical establishment represented by the A.G.M.F.

Two of the arrondissement medical associations in Paris, those of the Sixth and Sevenths arrondissements, voted against approval of Le Baron's syndicat. Dr. Généteix of the Sixth Arrondissment, wrote a summary of their views which was printed in *La France médicale,* the principal voice of the A.G.M.F. in Paris. These two arrondissement societies viewed the syndicat movement as unnecessary and dangerous. Génésteix remarked that the Union movement in general was indicative of the "deplorable" development of class warfare in the nation, of which doctors should not be a part. Unionization, in his eyes, would seriously damage the dignity of doctors, making them no better than "grocers, bell ringers and drapers." Syndicats, he believed, were appropriate for workers and small commercial men, but not for doctors whose "services could not be evaluated in terms of weight or wages." [34]

Généteix argued that perhaps syndicats were necessary for provincial doctors, but they were not needed in Paris. Généteix objected to the Union program to set tariff schedules, arguing that the fee charged a client was matter of the doctors' conscience and the client's pocket book. In the provinces, Généteix argued, a person's social and economic status were fairly obvious and known to all. In Paris, however, there was much hidden poverty and secret wealth, so only the habitual physician knew how much a person was truly worth, and should, moreover, not have to endure his brothers' scrutiny of what he was charging his clients. Génésteix also objected to Union's plan to create "black books" of patients who regularly did not pay their bills. These clients were then to be shunned by other doctors in the local syndicats. Généstiex felt such boycotting of patients by doctors would only create bad feeling between the public and doctors. [35]

Généteix pointed out that that doctors were not a homogeneous profession and did not all share the same professional interests. On these grounds he opposed the Union campaign against the abuses of doctors by insurance companies. In Généteix's mind this program should be undertaken by associations of the doctors who were employed by the companies. Further, Génésteix did not think it desirable to have a professional organization which, as the Union did, made membership open to all licensed doctors who paid dues and obeyed the syndicat by-laws and decisions. Généteix preferred organizations such as the Arrondissement societies and the governing board of the Paris-Seine associations, where all the members, he pointed out, were elected to the association and thus had intimate knowledge of the honorability and competence of each other. In Genesteix's eyes exclusive organizations with limited membership, typified by the Academy of Medicine and the A.G.M.F., could best pursue the doctors' professional interests. [36]

Promoters of the syndicats in Paris agreed with Généteix that all doctors did not share common interests. But they argued, contrary to Génésteix's view, that there was a group of Parisian physicians who needed the syndicat movement. These were the *médecins du quartier*, whom doctors in the Union movement saw as the urban counterparts of the provincial doctors who had started the syndicat movement. These neighborhood Paris doctors, they argued, were not adequately represented by the A.G.M.F. organizations which did nothing about the issues which most affected them, namely illegal practitioners and loss of patients to hospitals and dispensaries. [37]

Génésteix's comments were deemed worthy of a long rebuttal by Cézilly himself. Cézilly pointed out that if the Arrondissement societies had really taken up the professional issues they claimed to protect, the syndicat movement would not have been necessary. Cézilly charged that the arrondissement societies had steadily been losing members and were becoming increasingly ineffectual. [38] Cézilly defended tariff schedules which, he claimed, served the syndicats as guidelines rather than fixed rates. He reported that the schedules had helped to abolish the one-franc fee for doctors' visits in the provinces and therby raised the income of many poor country doctors by one-third. Cézilly noted that the Paris "princes of science" need not worry, the tariff schedules were not meant to apply to them. As for illegal practitioners, Cézilly agreed that they had little effect on the practices of the "rich and prestigious". However, they were a serious problem for the average practitioner, and made it difficult for young doctors to establish clienteles. [39]

The debate over syndicats became quite bitter and Union leaders often attacked the profession's traditional leaders in very harsh terms. They castigated those doctors who refused to join them, accusing them of being either too snobbish and selfish or too timid and weak. Non-jointers were accused of slavishly deferring to the elites. [40] This anti-establishment viewpoint was not limited to Paris practitioners but was heard throughout the syndicat movement. Members of the Rhône syndicat scorned the well-off doctors who refused to join them.

"As for the aristocrats of the profession, as for those who have a brilliant financial situation, due to their dazzling success and the favors of fate, they are indifferent to the issues of insurance societies, medical assistance, and conflicts over fees...As for the great masters of medical eduction in the hospitals and faculties, they should not forget the average practitioners, who were, after all, once their students, and who wage a daily battle for existence which is becoming more and more difficult." [41]

The opposition of some doctors of the Paris establishment and the A.G.M.F. to syndicalization did not do great harm to the Union movement. By 1902, the Seine syndicat had over nine hundred members. Its founder, Dr. Le Baron, became one of the leaders of the Union's fight against insurance societies, and became the first representative of the syndicats on the national council governing insurance societies. [42] Part of the reasons for the success of the syndicat movement was that in spite of their opposition to the profession's elites, Cézilly and his co-leaders had some important allies among those very elites. One of the most important was Dr. Paul-Camille-Hippolyte Brouardel (1837-1906) who played a critical role in solving the medical conflicts of the period.

Brouardel's career typified the background and connections of the medical elites. He took his doctorate at the Paris faculty and then rose through the hospital system to become a professor of legal medicine at the Paris Faculty of Medicine. In the 1880s, Brouardel reorganized morgue services in Paris and convinced officials of the importance of toxicology laboratories in identifying cause of death and aiding in criminal investigations. In 1881 he became a member of the Academy of Medicine and Dean of the Faculty of Medicine. In 1892, Brouardel was made a member of the Academy of Sciences. He also headed the *Annales d'hygiène et de médecine legale* and, along with Léon Bourgeois, and Waldeck-Rousseau, started the Permanent Extraparliamentary Anti-Tuberculosis Commission. He served on every important professional organization and bureaucratic committee in health care, and was the long-time president of the Comité consultatif d'Hygiène publique (C.C.H.P.). He was also a leading figure in the public health movement, a disciple of Louis Pasteur, and an important researcher in his own right. Brouardel's opinions carried a great deal of influence among legislators. He came to play a critical role in reconciling the professional goals of the Union movement and the changing attitudes of the medical establishment and state toward public health. Although he was sometimes at odds with the Union movement he realized its political potential and the necessity of supporting the goals of the private practitioners in order to gain their support for his own goals, the most important of which was the passing of public health legislation. Yet Brouardel himself also seems to have sympathized with the crisis felt by private practitioners and to have supported their quest to preserve private practice in the face of a new wave of state interest in medical care. [43]

When the doctors of *Le Concours* began their fight against the medical crisis they addressed three essential issues: the oversupply of doctors, the effects of illegal practice, and the worsening public image of doctors. In addition to alerting their readers to these problems, *Le Concours* immediately began to plan legislative solutions to them, including the rewriting of the law on the exercise of medicine and a plan for a medical assistance program to aid indigents in rural areas who were unable to afford the care of doctors.

The problem of overcrowding in the profession was an obsessive concern of doctors in the 1880s and 1890s. Page after page of *Le Concours* and the Union press was devoted to the issue. [44] Actually, as several authors have pointed out, the supply of doctors, measured as a ratio of doctors per inhabitants, reached a century high in the 1840s and had been decreasing ever since. [45] However, doctors at the end of the century had the impression that the ratio of inhabitants per doctor had reached its lowest level in their own time. This conclusion was based upon their own difficulties and that of their colleagues in finding clients. [46] The anxieties about oversupply were fueled by increased enrollments at medical schools and what doctors perceived to be increased utilization of illegal practitioners. This recourse to illegals may have been a real phenomenon: a reaction to the methods of the licensed practitioner of the era (see below).

Given the importance of the the overcrowding issue to the doctors of the Union movement, it is worthwhile to look closely at the statistics themselves. In appraising the number of practitioners and their relationship to the population, a distinction must be made between the two grades of licensed general medical practitioners, the *docteurs* and the *officiers de santé*. The *docteurs* were trained, examined and licensed by the faculties of medicine. Their training included courses, hospital experience, formal examinations and a thesis. The *officiers de santé* were created by the Law on the Practice of Medicine of 1805 as a corps of practitioners to replace the surgeons. The surgeons, whose vocation was abolished by the 1805 law, had supplied the major part of licensed general care in rural areas. The *officiers de santé* were intended to take over this role as it was felt that *docteurs* would be reluctant to practice in the backward, dull provinces. The *officiers* received generally two years of education at the departmental medical schools (which also trained pharmacists and midwives). *The officiers* did not write a thesis but underwent a period of apprenticeship to a *docteur*. At the end of this period they were examined and licensed by departmental medical juries.

From 1847 on there was a substantial increase in the number of *docteurs,* taking into consideration that between 1866 and 1876 there was a significant but temporary drop in their numbers due to the loss of the populations of Alsace and Lorraine. However, at the same time there was a drastic decrease in the number of *officiers de santé,* so that overall the number of practitioners, including both *docteurs* and *officiers* decreased between 1847 and 1876 (see Figure I-1). Measured as a ratio of practitioners to total population, there were significantly fewer practitioners available to the general public in 1876 than there had been in

1847 (see Table I-1). After 1876 the number of *officiers* continued its rapid decline, and the number of *docteurs* slowly increased, but the total number of practitioners available to the population remained relatively constant in the 1880s (see Figure I-2). After 1896, the number of practitioners available to the public finally began to increase for the first time since the 1840s. This increase was due to an increase in the number of *docteurs*. The fears about overcrowding, then, began at a time when the number of practitioners per population had been unchanged for some time, although after 1896 the anxiety of practitioners became more realistic.

Doctors were also upset by the increasing number of enrollments in medical schools in the 1890s. The number of diplomas issued each year for the medical doctorate had increased steadily from 590 in 1889 to 1,152 in 1901. [47] Doctors writing on the subject felt that two developments were responsible for the increased attractiveness of medical schools: the great publicity and prestige surrounding the scientific-medical advancements of the late nineteenth century, and changes in the educational system which made a secondary education available to a wider sector of the population. [48] One doctor complained that these changes meant that "young men of mediocre intelligence were entering the faculties of medicine." He predicted that the result would be that

"The son of the concièrge of the Faculty of Medicine is becoming a doctor, while the son of a doctor is reduced to the role of concièrge at the Faculty because the medical profession will become oversupplied with sons of concièrges." [49]

Other new developments made it easier for young would-be doctors to find a place in the Faculties. In 1870 there were only three faculties of medicine; in 1896 there were seven. [50] Doctors writing in the Union journals reported developments in science had affected medical education in a way that made it possible for more students to enter medical school. As the Faculties and medical schools began to require more training in science, they required less Latin and Greek; finally in 1885 the faculty in Paris did away with the classical baccalaureate as a requirement for entrance. [51]

The abolition of the *officers de santé* in 1892 also made it somewhat easier to pursue a doctorate in medicine. The *officiers* had recieved their training at the *Ecoles en plein exercise* and the *Ecoles préparatoires de Médecine et de Pharmacie.* [52] The abolition of the officiate naturally threatened the existence of these schools and educational authorities compensated by allowing the schools to take a greater role in the training of *docteurs.* Formerly students studying for the medical doctorate had been allowed to do a limited amount of their course work at the *Ecoles.* But after 1885, they could take some of their courses at the *Ecoles en plein exercise* and about three-quarters of them at the *Ecoles préparatoires.* The administrators of the provincial medical schools began to publicize the financial advantages of schooling at their insitutions where students could live at home or board in cities with generally lower costs of living than many of the locations of the Faculties. [53]

All of these factors contributed to a dramatic increase in the number of medical students after 1885. The number of students at the Paris Faculty reached a high of five thousand in 1894. As Dean of the Faculty, Brouardel began a campaign to discourage families from sending their sons into a medical career, warning them that due to overcrowding in the profession it would be very difficult to find clienteles or bureaucratic jobs after graduation. Pressure from Brouardel and from the Union was effective as the number of students at the Paris Faculty was down to four thousand in 1903. [54]

What the syndicat movement spoke of as a problem of too many practitioners was really a problem of distribution. The ratio of practitioners (including *docteurs* and *officiers de santé*) to population varied greatly between the departments and within individual departments (see Table I-2). Although cities certainly attracted a greater concentration of medical practitioners, urbanization alone does not adequately explain the distribution patterns of French physicians in the nineteenth century. Departments which were the locales of the faculties of medicine, such as Seine, Gironde and Hérault, not surprisingly, had large numbers of practitioners relative to their populations. However, some of France's major cities such as St. Etienne, Lyon, Brest and Nancy, were located in departments with relatively few practitioners. (see Table I-3). In the nineteenth century, departments undergoing rapid growth tended to have the fewest practitioners per inhabitants. [55] This might suggest that it took a certain period of time for the number of doctors to catch up to the population. However, cities like Paris and Marseille, which also were characterized by rapid population growth in the latter half of the nineteenth century, kept a steadily high rate of practitioners per population. It is more likely that the low medicalization rates in certain rapid growth areas is explained by the fact that industrial working class populations were not a very attractive clientele for doctors. Not only did workers have a difficult time paying medical fees but they tended to use hospitals and insurance societies to a greater extent than either the peasantry or the bourgeoisie. [56]

The highest concentration of practitioners per population was to be found in the south, in the Garonne Basin, Hérault, Pyrénées Orientales, Bouches-du-Rhône and the Var. [57] Several factors may explain this pattern. First of all after 1870 there were three faculties of medicine in this area, at Bordeaux, Montpellier and Toulouse, and a medical school at Marseille. In addition, at least until the 1890's, the economy of this area was relatively prosperous. Although not highly urbanized, the southwest was the locale of small, market-oriented family farms. Part of this area was characterized by what Maurice Agulhon has called the urban-village. [58] Finally, the coastal departments such as Herault and Pyrénées-Orientales possessed famous spas which attracted a heavy concentration of aristocratic and bourgeois health seekers and therefore many doctors as well.

It is evident that a certain standard of living was necessary to support the practice of doctors. Simple poverty may explain why doctors were not attracted to industrial areas or to bleak, backward rural areas like the Nivernais, Brittany, the Haute-Savoie and Hautes-Alpes. In spite of efforts to change it, particularly through the medical assistance program, the skewed distribution of doctors in France did not improve during the 1890s. The increase in doctors after 1896 did not help the distribution problem. Of the increase in doctors by 1031 between 1896-98, fifty-eight per cent constituted an increase in practitioners in urban areas which encompassed twenty-seven per cent of the population. Only forty-two per cent represented an increase in practitioners in rural areas which accounted for seventy-three per cent of the total population. [59]

In 1903 in many areas of the countryside there were still not nearly enough practitioners to reach all of the population. Of 36,000 communes, 29,000 (eighty-one per cent) had no *docteur* or *officier de santé;* and of 2,000 cantons, three hundred (fifteen per cent) had no *docteur* or *officier.* [60] At the same time that the pages of the professional press were full of articles on the problem of oversupply, there were also numerous advertisements from the mayors of rural villages, and from prefects and sub-prefects, advising young doctors of the need for a practitioner in a particular village or canton. [61] While recognizing that there was a great difference in the distribution of doctors throughout the nation, *Le Concours* still felt that overall there were too many doctors. [62]

Le Concours tended to publicize the high number of doctors in urban areas and ignore the lack of practitioners in rural areas. In the department of the Seine, the attractions of Paris produced the highest concentration of doctors in the nation. In 1881 there was already one practitioner per 1,414 and by 1896 the ratio had already fallen to one per 1,035 inhabitants. [63] *Le Concours* widely publicized this development in its continued commentary on over-crowding. The Union press also discussed the situation in several other areas which also underwent rapid increase in doctors at the same time, such as the Department of the Rhône where the number of doctors increased from 138 in 1881 to 295 in 1886. [64] Cézilly was greatly angered when the editor of *Le Figaro* proposed that the state sponsor a program to place one doctor in each commune. Cézilly called this idea ruinous to the medical profession.

Le Concours evaluated the proper number of clients per doctors as a function of the income they produced. In 1887 Cézilly argued the average clientele produced three to seven thousand francs a year, but that many practices only brought in only 1,200 to 2,500 francs a year. According to Cézilly, this was quite below what a doctor could live on decently. [65] As remedies for the perceived problem of "oversupply," *Le Concours* and the Union advocated making medical studies more difficult, exercising greater repression against illegal practice, and abolishing the *officiers de santé*. [66]

In the eyes of the Union movement, the effects of overcrowding in the profession greatly exacerbated the other general social, economic and professional problems which doctors faced. Doctors in the period generally felt that their economic status was deteriorating. The Union gave a great deal of publicity to an incident described in the Paris press of a young doctor who had been a "well-respected" student at the Paris

Faculty and ended up dead of starvation in the streets of Paris, allegedly because he was unable to find any clients. They cited this as a warning to parents and young people that France had too many doctors. [67] *Le Concours* drew attention to the families of deceased doctors who were left destitute after the death of their chief breadwinner and urged contributions to aid them. [68] Cézilly even suggested that the state should take on the responsibility of supporting the dependent survivors of doctors. [69] The elite medical journals also reported that some doctors were in desperate economic conditions and the Seine medical assocation indicated in 1893 that more and more doctors were applying to the A.G.M.F. for medical aid. [70]

Doctors claimed that part of their problem was due to increasing difficulties in securing payment from their clients. This in turn they blamed on changes in the relationship between doctor and patient. Within and without the syndicat movement, doctors in private practice felt that their public image had been greatly diminished in recent years. They seemed to believe there had been a "good old days," when families gave faithful patronage to one doctor whom they paid regularly and gladly. In these old good times, as doctors characterized it, the rich always added a little to their bills to make up for the free care the doctor gave to the poor; the bourgeoisie paid quickly and fully and considered their doctor a member of the family; workers and peasants paid what they could in goods and services and with their recognition and veneration. Doctors believed that by the end of the century the good old days had vanished: clients were generally lacking in respect and had become very lax in paying their bills. [71]

According to Brouardel, the antagonisms between doctors and the public had worsened in the last three decades of the nineteenth century. He based this perception largely on his long experience with medical issues in the courts, where he saw a growing trend toward more conflict between doctors and clients and more severity on the part of the courts in dealing with doctors. [72] Dr. Bach of the southern federation of syndicats (La Fédération médical, Toulouse) claimed that the "princes of science" in Paris were to blame for the loss of respect doctors generally felt. Bach said these elite doctors charged overly high fees and thus incurred the wrath of the public. [73] Many doctors also believed that the overcrowding of the profession had contributed greatly to this problem. They argued that the "struggle to survive" caused jealously and competition among doctors rather than cohesion damaging their public image. [74] Competition, according to this argument, forced doctors into dishonorable practices such as schemes with pharmacists to over-presecribe and receive kickbacks. [75] The result was that

"the medical corps in modern society has lost its influence; it no longer enjoys the respect and the sympathy that it formerly was surrounded with." [76]

Le Concours did not hesitate to report the nasty things said about doctors in the public press and to protest the complete unjustness of such statements. Dr. Greletty of Vichy regularly wrote articles in the society's journal protesting criticisms of doctors and praising their sacrifice and devotion. In this way Le Concours attempted to make doctors aware of public animosity, and it urged them not to be apathetic but to take the issue seriously and try to improve their image. [77] In opposition to the perceived public image of doctors as incompetent and greedy, *Le Concours* protrayed the private practitioner, especially the "médecin de campagne," as a tireless, devoted worker, enduring severe weather and desperate isolation to treat an ignorant, ungrateful, and often nonpaying clientele. [78]

The image campaign run by Grellety and others at *Le Concours* was an effort to promote a cerain idealized notion about the practice of medicine. According to Grellety's image, doctors performed a very valuable service, at a great personal cost in time and devotion, for which they were inadequately rewarded in terms of respect and financial compensation. Even Paul Brouardel, a scientific researcher, spoke of the relationship of physician and patient in a very broad and romantic fashion. In the eyes of Brouardel, the service which doctors performed was a subjective one. The doctor was the family confidant and advisor; his medical decisions were intertwined with his duty to promote the family interests. [79]

The Union movement also promoted the image of the doctor as family friend and advisor. Beyond this they made no examination of the services that doctors performed. *Le Concours* and the Union movement were essentially concerned with the general social image of the doctor. This image of devotion and sacrifice was the heart of their ideology. They used this ideology successfully to unite doctors in the Union movement; it was an ideology of social role rather than one of medical theory. The precise nature of the service which they performed was never defined and its usefulness was never questioned. As Freidson points out, the fact that the service performed by physicians is a consulting one that takes place in a one-to-one encounter between physician and client, makes it impregnable to outside examination and therefore to general criticism. As Freidson argues is true of doctors today, French doctors seemed very reluctant to look critically at their colleagues' methods. Doctors in the Union movement did not seem to be concerned over exactly what they and their colleagues were doing to cure the ills of their patients.

At the time that the medical sciences were being shaken by the developments in bacteriology, practitioners did not generally discuss its implications among themselves. Contrary to Freidson's observations, the adoption of bacteriological medicine as a coherent ideology was not an important factor in creating professional unity among doctors. The ideology of germ theory was important to the profession externally because it helped to legitimize the profession's goals in the public view. However, the ideology which united doctors internally in the Union movement was only a social image combined with common political and economic goals. The Union movement occurred at the very time when medical science was undergoing a radical transformation from the miasmatic theory of disease to germ theory and contagion. Among medical scientists in the academic world, this caused divisivness and hostility. [80] But doctors in the Union movement seemed hardly touched by these issues. In fact private practitioners were unified as never before due to their common social and political concerns.

The Union movement had some very straightforward ideas about how to solve the economic and image problems of doctors. Local syndicats made up basic tariff schedules to guide doctors in charging their clients. These schedules were usually made up in three levels, for workers and peasants, the middle classes, and the rich. The project to compile "black books," which Génésteix found so horrifying, was seriously promoted by the Union for a time but seems to have been dropped in the mid 1890s. But Doctors were told they had a right to be more aggressive in pursuing non-paying clients. *Le Concours* was particularly anxious to modify article 900 of the Civil Code, which under certain circumstances, prevented doctors from claiming bequests left them by clients. This article held that doctors, *officiers de santé,* midwives and pharmacists could not legally claim any bequests left them by clients whom they treated during a fatal illness unless the bequest was made prior to the onset of that illness. [81] *Le Concours* found this insulting as well as being sometimes a great financial loss, besides helping the doctors in his financial dealings with clients, the Union also had an impact on the fees paid by the state, as the following chapters will show.

As far as their relationships with one another were concerned, the Union urged doctors to work together and present a united front to the public. Doctors were told never to criticize one another, either on aspects of technique or personal issues, in front of the public. Such talk was to be kept among themselves. The Union also provided arbitration services to settle conflicts between doctors over clienteles or fees in order to keep them out of the civil courts and the public eye. The Union helped doctors to abritrate arrangements in the buying and selling of clienteles. The Union also prevented some doctors from selling clienteles, and then setting up practice again in the same area. [82]

The leaders of the Union emphasized that doctors should respect each other's territory of practice, defined in terms of a specific clientele or geographic area. *Le Concours* urged doctors not to make visits to rural patients residing in the area of practice of another doctor, even if the patients in question were not regular clients of the resident doctor. Cézilly complained that peasants frequently would send for a city doctor and ignore the physicians in their area, assuming that good doctors would never practice in the countryside areas. Cézilly urged that doctors called in to areas outside their usual practice first contact the local doctor and receive his blessing. Consultants, according to Cézilly, should always respect the prior rights of the resident doctors and encourage the locals to patronize their local physicians. General practitioners were urged to accompany consultants on their visits to the practitioners regular clients. [83]

The Union also tried to help doctors divide their clienteles more equitably when more than one rural practitioner practiced in the same area. An affair related by Cézilly illustrates that Union leaders could be effective in these matters. Upon returning to his native region to set up practice, a young medical school graduate faced the competition of a long-time practitioner who was the only médecin in the capital city of the arrondissement. The city had a population of 9,000, more than adequate to support two doctors; however, the resident practitioner held all the bureaucratic posts and would not pass on any clients to the young doctor. Since both doctors were members of *Le Concours,* the young doctor wrote to Cézilly to request his intercession.

Cézilly sent the established doctor a copy of his article on the problem of oversupply in which Cézilly urged estabished physicians to be generous in helping their younger colleagues. The young doctor later reported that Cézilly had convinced the resident doctor to share his clients and state posts with the young practitioner. Cézilly presented this story as a moral lesson to all doctors on collegiality. [84]

At the end of the century the Union movement formally became involved in deontology. [85] Deontological questions, matters relating to the professional relationships between doctors, had long been the terrain of the "grand masters" of medicine. By becoming involved in this issue, the leaders of the Union movement were quite aware that they were threatening the established elites. [86] Formerly deontology had not been specifically taught but only informally discussed with students by professors at the faculties. In the late 1890s, under the sponsorship of the Medical Society of the Twentieth Arondissement of Paris, Drs. Le Gendre and Leparge began to offer formal courses in deontology at the Paris faculty. [87]

The Union brought deontology outside the faculties to the average practitioner. Lead by Dr. Grasset, Union doctors created a national, and later international, Permanent Committee on Deontology. Grasset saw this as a counter to the traditional domination of deontology by the medical elites. He claimed that the "great masters" made dramatic pronouncements about the need for doctors to support one another only to contradict themselves by their own behavior. He accused some professors of providing examples by their own conduct which led their students to ridicule and scorn the "good practitioner." [88] When Grasset's committee had its first meeting in Paris, in July, 1900, they reported that the "great masters" stayed away. Grasset said he and his associates were quite content that the elites had thus excluded themselves from regulating deontology for the bulk of the profession. [89] Grasset introduced new subjects to the subject of deontology. Besides a more explicit treatment of financial and clientele conflicts, they also used the deontological committee to fight against insurance societies by putting pressure on young doctors not to take positions with such organizations. [90]

The problem of illegal practitiones was the single most important issue to doctors of the Union movement. In the late nineteenth century, traditional, nonlicensed medical practitioners such as bonesetters, urine readers, and herbalists were still common in rural areas. Their practice was illegal under the 1805 law, but they were rarely prosecuted to any effective extent. Illegal practice was tied up with all the other problems of which doctors complained. According to the private practitioners, illegals took away patients and made it difficult for doctors to practice in certain rural areas. Furthermore, they argued that the existence of illegals diminshed the prestige and value of medical degrees. As Cézilly explained, in many areas patients preferred charlatans to licensed practitioners:

"The peasant does not call a doctor until after exhausting the
arsenal of charlatanism.--He calls the doctor to find out what he
is going to die of. He takes care to stipulate that the doctor
should not return unless he is called for, and that call never
comes, unless it is to attest to the cause of death." [91]

Doctors often complained that charlatans, including bonesetters,
urine readers, sorcerers, spiritualists, nuns, herbalists, as well as pharmacists and midwives who overstepped the bounds of their license, were
often more popular than doctors in rural communities. [92] One doctor
claimed that he disguised himself as an illegal practitioner in a rural
community and found he had many more patients than as a licensed
practitioner. [93] Religious healers were especially popular in some areas.
In 1902 a farm worker in the mountains around St. Etienne, who
claimed to be called by heaven to be a healer, reportedly had a steady
lineup of clients at his mountain hut, coming from Saint Etienne,
Roanne, Puy, Vienne and Lyon. He was known in the mountain region
as "Saint Barkari." Prosecution, conviction, and a fifty-franc fine from
authorities only enhanced his popularity and his clientele. [94] Although
the problem of illegal practitioners plagued doctors throughout the
nineteenth century, doctors of the 1880s and 1890s widely believed that
the patronage of illegal practitioners was increasing. Again, they made
such pronoucements while conjuring up images of a better past when
doctors had everywhere enjoyed respect. [95]

But their notion of more patronage of illegals may have reflected a
reality. There is no evidence that doctors were any more effective

against illness than the illegals. Moreover, some techniques used in licensed practice were harmful and unpleasant. Léonard and Freidson have suggested that the increased patronage of illegals may have become more widespread around the middle of the century as a result of techniques doctors were using at this time. [96] Some of the remedies used by doctors were very simple, of the sort that a good housewife and certainly any herbalist might use. These included teas and infusions used for cholera and fever. But even in the 1890s, doctors were still using techniques and medicines of questionable efficacy. Not a few of these must have been very unpleasant and even quite harmful. [97] Purging and bleeding were still in use around 1890, although it was recognized that bleeding, in general, was a dangerous practice. Doctors realized it was one of the techniques that had caused the public to be wary of their services. [98] However, in 1879 bleeding was still recommended for cases of cerebral hemorrhage, if the patient was formerly strong and robust. [99] In 1892, bleeding still appeared on tariff schedules. [100] It was also recognized that purging of the stomach could bring on hemorrhage; however in 1892 purging was still frequently recommended as a remedy against a variety of digestive complaints, from mild indigestion to intestinal lesions. [101]

New technical developments and scientific discoveries did not necessarily have good consequences for patients. Electricity was a popular treatment at the end of the nineteenth century, as it had been at the end of the eighteenth. It was recommended for a variety of conditions, including paralysis, anemia, pale skin, and chorea. [102] Electric shock was particularly popular for gynecological and obstetric problems. Direct application of electric current to the uterus was used in the care of post-partum hemorrhage. One doctor recommended "electrical baths" if this failed. [103] Direct application of electric current to the uterus was also recommended for hysteria, melancholy, fibroid tumors, vaginal lesions and abdominal swelling. [104] Bacteriological theory did not always have positive results either: some doctors carried the notion of disinfection to an extreme, suggesting it was helpful in certain cases to "disinfect" organs of the body. Again, the stomach and female reproductive organs were the target. Strong antiseptic solutions were used; in one treatment the solution was so caustic that the doctor recommended the conjunctive use of cocaine. [105]

Given the practitioners' overwhelming concern with keeping clients, why would they use such extreme measures even when it was clear that they distressed the patient and might drive them to unlicensed practitioners using more gentle techniques? Freidson explaines that drastic techniques are encouraged by the doctor's need to present some tangible evidence of his intervention. Freidson also points out that the ways in which the expertise is defined in the medical profession demands that the doctor do something in the face of disease. Freidson explains that the doctor is called as a result of the helplessness and bewilderment of the client, with the assumption that the doctors will understand a phenomenon which ordinary people cannot. In order to prove his expertise, the physician feels compelled to take some action. [106] Further, as Larson points out, the encounter of patient and doctor is one where exchange is involved. [107] The doctor is paid for his services and the patient expects some concrete evidence that a service has been performed. These pressures, according to Larson, could cause doctors to take some action which because of its extreme nature would be a testament of the doctor's ability to act. It is apparent that in the last half of the nineteenth century this need to demostrate intervention was strong enough, at times, to override the need to keep clients. This seems to have driven clients away from doctors and into the arms of the more gentle care of herbalists, urine readers, patent medicine sellers, and wise-women.

In its publications and meetings, the Union movement did not pay much attention to medical techniques or to the effect which various techniques had on maintaining or repelling clients. The doctors' major concern was to tighten up their monopoly on practice through new legislation on the practice of medicine. They believed that new legislation was necessary because their terrain of practice was being threatened not only by illegal practitioners but also by the new directions in medical care indicated by the bacteriological revolution.

Elite doctors and the average practitioner had quite different points of view about the impact of the public health movement on the private practitioners, but all agreed that the practice of medicine was changing. It was clearly recognized that the bacteriological revolution might dramatically transform the role of the doctor. There was considerable discussion that medicine had become preventative as well as palliative. As Dr. F. Ranse, editor of the *Gazette Médical de Paris* observed in

1889:

"Formerly the doctor's terrain did not go beyond the limits of the family. Today the role of the doctor has been extended considerably. The revolution in medicine from microbion doctrines has caused public health to take wings....The result is that for the first time the physician has a true social role to fill....The old 'family doctor' has become the guardian of the public health, the 'public doctor'". [108]

The transformation of the practice of medicine from a palliative to a preventative role was seen to enlarge greatly the doctor's role in society.

What was the relationship of the syndicat movement to the bacteriolgical revolution? The prevention function, doctors recognized, belonged in the realm of public health activity. Union doctors agreed with observers such as Ranse, that new functions were expected of doctors as a result of the public health movement. Doctors were now expected to practice asepsis and antisepsis, which as Cézilly pointed out, took time and required extra expense. They were expected to educate the public in matters of hygiene, identify sources of contagion, and generally lead the hygiene movement. However, the Union movement complained that all of these new duties were expected of them with no compensation. Moreover, it was widely believed that the number of the sick had been reduced by advancements in hygiene, thus aggravating the practical difficulties for doctors created by an overcrowded profession. Rarely did a doctor note that in reality the opposite might be true: the notion of infection and the growing public awareness of microbes was causing people to seek medical care more and more frequently. [109] On the contrary, the refrain most often heard among doctors was "more doctors, fewer patients." [110] Thus in the eyes of the Union movement, the bacteriological revolution contributed to the medical crisis. Doctors were being impoverished by the ever increasing competition for fewer patients, and they were being expected to perform new duties with no pay.

The bacteriological revolution brought another threat to private practitioners through the increased utilization of hospitals and the creation of new kinds of institutional care. Hospitals in France, from the time of the Revolution, were under the control of the state through the public assistance bureaucracy. After 1888, the hospitals were under the control of the reorgan.zed C.S.A.P. (*Conseil supérieur d'Assistance publique.)* Historically, hospitals were only patronized by the destitute and homeless; even the very poor avoided them unless they were totally without resources. In the late nineteenth century, however, hostpitals were becoming less feared by the lower classes and increasingly utilized by the middle classes. Critical private practitioners noted that some hospitals were even becoming "luxurious". [111] According to private practitioners such developments helped the pocketbooks and careers of the hospital surgeons to their own detriment. [112] Hospital patients passed out of the hands of the private practitioner because hospitals were staffed separately, mostly by the elites of the educational establishment and their students. Two critical private practitioners stated the matter very clearly: "when patients go to the hospital, they are lost to us." [113]

Doctors of the Union movement were incensed that the rich were abusing hospital care while the elite doctors who staffed and administered the hospitals did nothing to prevent such abuse. [114] Doctors were also concerned about the treatment of working class and middle class patients, free of charge, at the hospitals and their attached clinics. These attached clinics offered free consultations by members of the Academy of Medicine, chiefs of the Paris hospital staffs, and professors at the Paris Faculty of Medicine. This was the standard practice at the other faculties of medicine and their hospitals throughout the nation. [115] This problem was made worse with the appearance of neighborhood dispensaries and clinics which welcomed the middle classes for slight fee, much below that charged by the neighborhood practitioner. [116] Private doctors in the cities had long been envious of the clients lost to the free care offered at the faculty hospitals and clinics, now this situation was being worsened by the building of neighborhood clinics and dispensaries. [117] Syndicat doctors complained that "petite bourgeois, rentiers, fonctionnaires," were all abusing free care at the hospitals and clinics, and that clinic doctors were continuing to follow the progress of their patients through home visits, giving out free medication, bandages and similar medical materials. [118]

The doctors who worked at the hospitals did not receive high salaries. However, such positions were quite prestigious and were paths to lucrative government posts. More importantly, they brought the fame and respect necessary to attract a well-paying bourgeois and aristocratic clientele in private practice. Hospital interns received training and a chance to enter the elites, if they succeeded in sufficiently impressing their mentors. Private pracitioner complained that young doctors in the hospitals gained prestige that they were too inexperienced to really deserve. [119] Thus hospitals, their privileged staff, and the free care they offered, were a long-time grievance to private practitioners.

The academic elites saw hospital services as a useful training milieu and a way for young doctors to establish their reputation. They believed that the syndicat leaders exaggerated the problem of abuse of free clinic and dispensary care by bourgeois clients. They also felt that attempts to regulate this would be an affront to the liberty of patients and doctors. Moreover, it would hurt the young hospital doctors to deny them the experience of relating to a wide variety of patients. [120] The syndicate doctors, in contrast, saw hospitals as a threat to all doctors. In their minds, hospitals made it difficult for young private practitioners to find a clientele. They felt that eventually the dispensaries and the increased utilization of hospitals by the bourgeoisie would destroy the private prctitioners of the cities. [121]

The battle against hospitals, dispensaries and clinics was one of the strongest efforts of the Union movment. This effort can be seen in many of the important medical reforms in which the Union was involved in the era; most notably the Medical Assistance Program. The Union always attempted to deny the necessity of hospitalization, arguing that isolation of contagious patients and the creation of germ-safe environments, could be managed in the patient's home. The Union even tried to argue that most surgery should be done at the patient's home. [122] The Union did admit that the hospital had some useful functions. It recognized that the hospital was the learning ground of young doctors and the experimental terrain of science. [123] The poor were seen as the proper subjects of scientific research. As one critic put it, the poor were more "docile," would allow themselves to be examined "without a murmur," and would submit to medical techniques which were difficult to experiment with on clients in an ordinary practice. This writer went on to suggest that the best way to keep middle class and working class patients away from the clinics was to schedule consultation hours during times when it would be inconvenient for workers or those with business interests to attend. Further, he recommended that all examinations be done out in the open, so that middle class clients would be too embarrassed to be seen. Apparently the poor either were not thought to care about such matters or had no alternatives. [124] The Union doctors argued that while treatment of the poor in hospitals was necessary and even desireble, hospital administration should put tighter controls on who was cared for. Further, they argued that hospitals should stop expanding their staffs. [125]

The battle against increased hospital care was only a part of a larger issue for doctors in the Union movement. This was the general problem of state involvement in medical care. French doctors had long feared that they would all eventually become state civil servants. As far back as the 1845 Doctors' Congress private physicians were determined to fight the spread of *fonctionnairisme*. However, the attitude of doctors toward positions in the bureaucracy was ambivalent. Those doctors without such posts criticized the advantages of those who held them and resented the favoritism shown by appointing officials. However, in fact most doctors eagerly sought such part-time public posts as inspector for needy children's services, school inspector, and cantonal physicians. These jobs gave them much needed added income and more importantly, carried with them the official benedication of the state, thus anointing the doctor with the prestige necesary to attract a larger clientele. Brouardel noted that there were over sixty applicants for the job of doctor-assistant to the Prefecture of Police in Paris, although the salary was only six hundred francs a year. [126] The prestige of government posts explains why doctors were willing to take on nonpaying appointments such as epidemic doctor, and membership on arrondissement and department hygiene councils. Because such civil service positions were usually only part-time occupations, requiring perhaps only a few days a year of service, *médecins-fonctionnaires* enjoyed the best of both worlds: the security, prestige, and some economic benefits of a government job, plus a private practice, enhanced by the status of government position. Further, such positions put the doctor in close contact with prefects, subprefects, and public assistance administrators, and increased the chances of gaining other lucrative positions or being called on to provide official assistance in criminal cases. Court cases were especially beneficial because of the publicity they brought to a participating doctor. Thus, in spite of the opposition to *fonctionnairisme* expressed in the 1840s, the number of these posts increased greatly during the Second Empire and Third Republic. Brouardel observed that *fonctionnairisme* was a devisive force among doctors, damaging the internal solidarity of the profession. [127] The regular doctors in private practice, outside of the privileged circle, resented these elite physicians who dominated bureaucratic posts, but hoped also to gain such positions themselves.

In the 1890s, as bureaucrats were making plans to expand public health and assistance services, doctors were very alarmed about the accompanying threat of more *fonctionnairisme*. The Union movement became determined to oppose the spread of any state intervention which would mean the maintainance of this old hierarchy. The syndicat insisted that two of its own great virtues were its independence of public powers and its determination to resist the increase of the power of the medical and public health buraucracy. [128] In this era of the Panama scandal and Dreyfus affair, some writers linked medical anti-fonctionnairisme with anti-semitism. An article appearing in one of the major Paris professional journals in 1900 quoted antisemitic leader Drumont in arguing that the interventionism of the state in medical affairs was a result of growing Jewish control of the state and society. [129]

In 1900, in a survey made by the journal *Le Concours,* among its subscribers asking for solutions to the problems of oversupply, one writer suggested that the only answer was for doctors to resign themselves to all becoming civil servants, since that was the direction in which the medical system was evolving. Cézilly, however, strongly objected. "No, we must never give in to this pessimism, but continue to fight oversupply through our own independent means." [130] The term "independent", however, did not mean that Union doctors would seek total autonomy from the state. While fighting for the medical system of liberal-private practice and the establishment of a professional mono-poly, state action would in fact become the doctors' greatest weapon.

The Union movement became a powerful lobby on behalf of private doctors. The unprecedented unity of doctors which the movement achieved was due to several factors. The movement's leaders promoted a vague but persuasive image of the doctors' role in society which could attract large numbers of doctors while covering up their doctrinal and practical differences. The Union provided pragmatic services such as insurance and legal protection as well as a means of dealing with deontological problems. And probably of greatest importance, through a variety of means the Union provided doctors with some solutions to their economic difficulties.

The Union movement was dedicated to preserving the principle of medical care through private contract between doctor and client. General practitioners in the syndicats saw this as crucial to their well-being. Securing their monopoly over medical practice meant the continuation and extension of this system of medical care in opposition to institutional care either in the form of hospitals or dispensaries. The relationship of the syndicat movement to the bacteriological revolution was, therefore, ambiguous. On one hand, the Union leaders saw many of the developments in hospital care and public health as a threat, on the other hand, the Union was quite willing to take advantage of the new prestige of the medical sciences to promote the professional interests of physicians.

Figure I-1
Docteurs, Officiers de Santé, and Total Practitioners
in France, 1847-1906.

Key: /// = Total practitioners
       *** = Docteurs
       +++ = Officiers de Santé

Numbers in thousands
0   1   2   3   4   5   6   7   8   9   10   11   12   13   14   15   16   17   18
Year

1847   18099
//
******************************** 10643
++++++++++++++++++++++++++ 7456

1866
/// 16822
******************************** 11254
+++++++++++++++++ 5568

1876
// 14376
******************************** 10743
+++++++++++ 3633

1881
// 14973
********************************** 11643
+++++++++++ 3203

1886
/// 14789
********************************** 11995
+++++++++ 2794

1891
// 14969
************************************** 12407
++++++++ 2512

1896
/// 15017
** 13412
+++++ 1605

Figure I-1
Docteurs, Officier de Santé, and Total Practitioners
in France, 1847-1906.
(continued)

Key: /// = Total practitioners
        *** = Docteurs
        +++ = Officiers de Santé

Numbers in thousands
0 1 2 3 4 5 6 7 8 9 10 11 12 13 14 15 16 17 18
Year
1901   17108
//
** 15907
+++++ 1201

1906   19136
//
                                                            18211
****
+++ 928

Figure I-2.
Docteurs, Officiers de Santé, and Total Practitioners
per population in France
1847-1906

One practitioner per: (in thousands)
above 25,000

```
                                                    +        +

24                                          +

23

22
 .
 .
 .
14                                      +

13

12

11

10                      +

9

8

7           +

6

5  +

4  *        *
                         *
3            X          X*        X*
        X                             X*
2  X                                         X*

1

   1847    1866    1876    1886    1896  1901   1906
```

Key: Total Practitioners/population = X
          Docteurs/population = *
          Officiers de Santé/population = +

Table I-1
Practitioners Per Population in France
1847-1906

Year	Population	Officiers de Santé	Officiers/ Population. One per:	Docteurs	Docteurs/ Population One per: (Docteurs)	Total Practitioners (Officiers and Docteurs)	Total Practitioners/ Population. One per:
1847	35,470,000[1]	7,456[2]	4,757	10,643[2]	3,333	18,099[2]	1,959
1866	38,080,000	5,568	6,839	11,254	3,384	16,822	2,264
1876[5]	36,830,000	3,633	10,137	10,743	3,428	14,376	2,562
1886	38,230,000	2,794[3]	13,683	11,995[3]	3,187	14,789[3]	2,585
1896	38,520,000	1,605	24,000	13,412	2,872	15,017	2,565
1901	38,980,000	1,201[4]	32,456	15,907[4]	2,450	17,108[4]	2,278
1906	39,267,000	928	42,313	18,211	2,156	19,136	2,052

1 Annuaire Statistique de la France, 1930, pp 11-12.

2 Recueil des Travaux du Commitée Consultatif d'hygiène Publique de la France, V. 16 (1886), pp 124-125.

3 Annuaire Statistique de la France V. 18, pp 510-511.

4 Ibid., V. 44, pp 34-37.

5 Drop in population and practitioners reflects the loss of Alsace and Lorraine.

Table I-2
Density of <u>Officier</u> de <u>santé</u>, <u>Docteurs</u>,
and Total Practitioners by Department
in 1896 [1]

Department (by region)	Officiers de Santé one per:	Docteurs one per:	Total Practitioners (Docteurs and Officiers) one per:
<u>NORD</u>			
Nord	11,184	4,017	2,955
<u>ARTOIS-PICARDIE</u>			
Pas-de-Calais	7,192	6,382	3,381
Somme	4,359	5,732	4,359
<u>NORMANDIE</u>			
Calvados	13,905	3,659	2,897
Eure	16,221	3,548	2,911
Manche	62,506	4,032	3,788
Orne	42,395	3,570	3,292
Seine-Inférieure	18,618	3,419	2,889
<u>BRETAGNE</u>			
Finistère	92,456	9,020	8,218
Côtes-du-Nord	30,803	7,247	5,867
Ille-et-Vilaine	9,147	4,573	3,049
Loire-Inférieure	17,949	3,047	2,605
Morbihan	48,636	8,230	7,039
<u>REGION-PARISIENNE</u>			
Aisne	12,309	3,735	2,865
Eure-et-Loir	31,163	3,505	3,151
Oise	11,897	3,236	2,544
Seine-et-Marne	39,893	2,720	2,546
Seine-et-Oise	33,454	2,151	2,021
<u>SEINE</u>			
Seine	35,140	1,067	1,035

[1] Dr. Maurice Lésieur, <u>Répertoire officiel de la
Médicine et de la Pharmacie français</u>, 1896.

Table I-2
Density of Officier de Santé, Docteurs,
and Total Practitioners by Department
in 1896 (continued)

Department (by region)	Officiers de Santé one per:	Docteurs one per:	Total Practitioners (Docteurs and Officiers) one per:
ALSACE-LORRAINE			
Meurthe-et-Moselle	5,552	2,915	1,911
Meuse	145,192	3,376	3,299
Haut-Rhin (Belfort)	0	8,004	8,004
Vosges	210,706	3,975	3,901
CHAMPAGNE			
Ardennes	28,987	3,751	3,321
Aube	62,858	2,703	2,592
Marne	12,559	2,990	2,415
Haute-Marne	58,014	2,937	2,795
LOIRE-MOYENNE			
Indre-et-Loire	17,740	2,762	2,390
Loir-et-Cher	21,396	4,031	3,392
Loiret	46,377	2,728	2,576
Maine-et-Loire	17,162	3,279	2,753
PLAINES-DU-CENTRE			
Allier	60,625	2,411	2,319
Cher	115,908	4,458	4,292
Indre	41,315	3,908	3,570
Nièvre	111,299	3,552	3,442
Vienne	18,784	3,596	3,018
PERCHE-ET-MAINE			
Mayenne	29,198	4,588	3,965
Sarthe	53,134	3,795	3,542

Table I-2
Density of Officier de Santé, Docteurs,
and Total Practitioners by Department
in 1896 (continued)

Department (by region)	Officiers de Santé one per:	Docteurs one per:	Total Practitioners (Docteurs and Officiers) one per:
MASSIF-CENTRAL			
Cantal	29,297	3,720	3,301
Corrèze	35,821	3,582	3,256
Creuse	23,280	4,232	3,581
Haute-Loire	105,566	7,197	6,738
Lozère	132,151	4,719	4,556
Puy-de-Dôme	20,558	2,734	2,413
Hautes-Vienne	26,837	3,833	3,354
BOURGOGNE			
Côte-d'Or	40,907	2,438	2,301
Haute-Saône	22,740	3,790	3,248
Saône-et-Loire	155,309	3,956	3,858
Yonne	27,721	2,501	2,294
REGION-LYONNAISE			
Loire	156,334	5,254	5,084
Rhône	139,888	2,197	2,163
PLANES-DU-RHONE			
Ardèche	90,875	6,731	6,267
Drôme	33,721	3,746	3,372
JURA			
Ain	70,313	3,906	3,700
Doubs	23,234	3,319	2,904
Jura	53,228	3,802	3,548
ALPES			
Basses-Alpes	9,845	3,193	2,411
Hautes-Alpes	22,645	5,959	4,717
Isère	23,705	3,896	3,346

Table I-2
Density of Officier de Santé, Docteurs,
and Total Practitioners by Department
in 1896 (continued)

Department (by region)	Officiers de Santé one per:	Docteurs one per:	Total Practitioners (Docteurs and Officiers) one per:
GASCOGNE			
Gers	5,329	2,003	1,456
Landes	8,882	2,396	1,887
BORDELAIS			
Gironde	20,247	1,853	1,697
ACQUITAINE			
Aveyron	64,910	3,573	3,386
Dordogne	35,755	2,834	2,626
Lot	48,080	2,861	2,701
Lot-et-Garonne	22,285	2,557	2,294
BAS-LANGUEDOC			
Aude	19,407	2,020	1,837
Gard	9,675	2,811	2,178
Hérault	22,365	1,752	1,625
HAUT-LANGUEDOC			
Ariège	18,303	3,600	3,008
Haute-Garonne	7,920	1,882	1,521
Tarn	42,478	2,594	2,444
Tarn-et-Garonne	25,048	2,636	2,385
PROVENCE			
Bouches-du-Rhône	6,738	1,684	1,347
Var	14,723	2,453	2,103
Vaucluse	13,128	2,813	2,316
Alpes-Maritime	6,676	1,065	919
OUEST MARITIME			
Charente	44,529	3,152	2,944
Charente-Inférieure	45,345	2,222	2,118
Deux-Sèvres	41,790	5,600	4,938
Vendée	20,078	3,775	3,177

Table I-2 /
Density of Officier de Santé, Docteurs,
and Total Practitioners by Department
in 1896 (continued)

Department (by region)	Officiers de Santé / one per:	Docteurs one per:	Total Practitioners (Docteurs and Officiers) one per:
PYRENEES /			
Basses-Pyrénees	14,605	2,680	2,265
Hautes-Pyrénees	5,340	2,280	1,598
Pyrenées-Orientales	8,682	2,935	2,193
SAVOIE			
Savoie	86,596	3,711	3,558
Haute-Savoie	53,174	4,923	4,506

Table I-3
Medical Density in 1881 for Departments Containing Areas
With the Greatest Rates of Urban Growth in the
Nineteenth Century [1]

One practitioner per:

Meurthe-et-Moselle (Nancy)	6,258
Finistère (Brest)	5,587
Loire (St. Étienne)	5,502
Rhône (Lyons)	5,148
Isère (Grenoble)	3,559
Aube (Troyes)	3,191
Nord (Lille)	2,730
Haute-Vienne (Limoges)	2,646
National Average	2,534
Marne (Rheims)	2,510
Var (Toulon)	1,989
Bouches-du-Rhône (Marseille)	1,574
Haute-Garonne (Toulouse)	1,541
Seine (Paris)	1,294

[1] Hugh D. Clout, "Urban Growth 1500-1900," in
Hugh D. Clout, ed. Themes in the Historical Geography
of France, 1975.

NOTES TO CHAPTER I

1. Crisis was a term the doctors themselves used, repeatedly, to describe their own situation: See for example: "Dr. Thierry, "Considerations sur les causes de la crise médicale actuelle," *Bulletin des Sociétés médicales d'Arrondissement,* (hereinafter Bul. des Soc. méd. d'Arron)., V. 3, N. VII, (April 5, 1900), p 268; Dr. Duchesne, "Quelques rémarques sur la crise médicale," *Bulletin des Syndicats médicaux de France* (hereinafter, Bul. des Syn. med. de France), (Oct. 1900) p 980.

2. Sussman and Weisz.

3. Sussman, Sussman does not take adequate note of the complaints on the part of some doctors against *fonctionnairisme* which would indicate the neo-corporist, or pro-state-interventionist stance was not shared by all doctors. This issue would be made more clear if Sussman had appraoched the 1845 period from the standpoint of a split in the profes-sional between elites and average practitioners and their professional goals.

4. My biographical source for Cézilly is his ardent admirer and fellow syndicalist, J. Noir. Noit wrote a short biography upon the occasion of Cézilly's death. He does not discuss Cézilly's educational background at all. This suggests that his backround was very humble and that he

possibly did not attend a faculty but became a *docteur* through a provincial medical school and his navy service.

5. J. Noir, "Auguste Cézilly", *Bulletin Official des syndicats médicaux de France,* (hereinafter, Bul. Off. des syn. méd. de France), N. 21 (Nov. 5, 1902), p 446.

6. *Gazette Hebdomadaire des Sciences médicales de Bordeaux,* V. 13, N. 7, (Feb. 14, 1892) p 82; all translations are my own.

7. J. Noir, *Ibid,* p 445.

8. Dr. A. Cézilly, "A Nos Adherents," *Le Concours médical,* (hereinafter: Le Concours), V. 1, N. 1, (July 5, 1879). p 2.

9. "A Nos Adherents," *Le Concours,* V. 1, N. 1, (July 5, 1879). p 1; A. Cézilly, "Aux Membres du Concours," *Le Concours* V. 10, N. 1, (Jan. 7, 1888), p 1.

10. The first decade of *Le Concours* has been described by Jacques Léonard in "Les Débuts du 'Concours médical'", *Histoire des Sciences médicales,* Vol. VIV, N. 4, (1980) p 453-58.

11. Dr. Gassot, "Historique de la Société du Concours médical," (Bul. des syn des Méd. de France, N. 37 (1889). pp 322-323.

12. Dr. J. Noir, *Ibid,* Dr. Gassot, *Ibid.*

13. J. Noir, *Ibid.*

14. Dr. Gassot, "Historique de la Société du Concours médical," *Bul. des Syn. méd de Fr.,* N. 31, (1889), p 323.

15. Dr. Mignen, "Il faut organiser de nouveaux syndicats," *Le Concours*, V. 13, N. 5, (Jan. 31, 1897); Cézilly, *Le Concours*, V. 14, N. 15, (April 9, 1892), pp 169-171. Versions of exactly when and by whom the syndicat movement was founded conflict somewhat, especially between Mignen's, Noir's and Cézilly's, I have chosen to rely on Mignen and Cézilly because they were personally involved.

16. Dr. Paul Brouardel, *La Profession médicale au commencement du siècle*, 1903, pp 226-230; "Nécrologie, M. le Dr. Fourmestreaux, *Bul. Off. de l'Union des Syn. méd. de France*, V. 16, N. 11 (June 5, 1902)

17. Dr. J. Noir, *Ibid.*

18. Dr. A. Cézilly, "A Nos Adherents," *Le Concours*, V. A, N. a, (July 5, 1879), p 2.

19. Dr. F. de Ranse, "Commentaire de la Nouvelle Loi sur l'Exercise de la Médecine," *Gazette médicale de Paris*, Series 7, V. VIII, N. 23, p 267.

20. See Chapters IV and V.

21. "Les syndicats médicaux," *Gazette médicale de Liège*, V. 5, N. 4, (Oct. 27, 1892). pp 37-40, Belgan doctors followed the French syndicalization movement closely, and publicized its successes as a way of stimulating their own movement.

22. Dr. Mignen, "Il faut organiser de noveaux syndicats," *Le Concours*, V. 13, N. 5 (Jan. 31, 1891). Brouardel estimated 120 member syndicats in 1903: Brouardel, *La Profession médicale*, P 226.

23. Corbeil, Etampes, Pontoise, Rambouillet, Versaille (Arrondissement not city).

24. "Listes des Syndicats adherents à l'Union," *Bul. de l'Union des syn. méd. de Fr.*, (Jan, 1893): List of member syndicats included the departments of, Aisne, Algerie, Ardèche-et-Drome (one combined syndicat of the Valley of the Rhône, centered at Tournon), Ardennes (3 syndicats), Aube, Bouches-du-Rhône (2), Calvados, Charente, Charente-Inférieure, Cher, Corrèze, Corse, Eure (2), Finistére (2), Gard, Gironde (2), Haute-Saône, Indre-et-Loire, Isére, Loire-Inférieure, Marne, Mayenne, Nord (2), Oise, Orne (2), Pas-de-Calais, Sarthe (2), Seine-et-Oise (5), Seine-Inférieure, Vendée, Vienne.

25. at Avesnes and Douai.

26. See chapter V.

27. See chapters IV and V.

28. Brouardel, *Ibid,* p 223. The A.G.M.F. actually descended from the *l'Association des médecins de la Seine,* founded in 1833, and still a part of the A.G.M.F. in this period.

29. Lyon médical, N. 14, April 5, 1891.

30. Brouardel, *La Profession médicale,* pp 222-225.

31. Cézilly, "Les syndicats médicaux à Paris," *Le Concours,* V. 14, N. 12, (Mar 19, 1892), pp 140-143; *La France médicale et Paris médicale* (hereinafter, La France médicale), V. 39, N. 9, (Feb. 26, 1892), P. 138.

32. Dr. Lannelongue was elected president of the A.G.M.F. in 1892, upon the death of Dr. H. Roger. Lannelongue was formerly on the

governing board of the Seine-Paris Arrondissement Associations: "l'Association générale des médecins de France," *La France médicale* V. 39, N. 18, (April 29, 1892), p 273.

33. It is interesting to note that the founders of the Seine syndicat turned the word "syndicat" into an adjective, and framed it with the words "Association" and "professionnelle." The older groups in other areas were usually simply called "Syndicat médicaux.." or "Syndicat des médecins..".

34. Dr. Génésteix, Société médicale du VIe Arrondissement, "l'Association syndicale professionnelle des médecins de la Seine," *La France médicale,* V. 39, N. 3, (Feb. 26, 1892), pp 138-144.

35. *Ibid.*

36. *Ibid.*

37. *Ibid.*

38. Cézilly "Les syndicats médicaux à Paris," *Le Concours,* V. 14, N. 12, (Mar. 19, 1892), pp 140-43.

39. *Ibid.*

40. Dr. R. Millon, "La Bonne parole," *Bul. Off. de l'Union des Syn. méd. de France,* N. 2 (Jan. 20, 1902), pp 23-34.

41. *Bulletin du Syndicat de l'Association des Médecins du Rhône,* V. 1, N. 1, (May 1, 1901), p 9.

42. "Nécrologie de M. de Dr. J. Le Baron," *Bul. Off. de l'Union des Syn. méd. de France,* N. 2 (Jan. 20, 1902), pp 23-34.

43. Horace Bianchon, *Nos Grandes médecins d'aujourd'hui.* 1891, pp 39-44; *Histoire générale de la médecine,* p 443.

44. The issue of oversupply of practitioners was an old one. Complaints on this score were heard as early as the Restoration period: Jacques Léonard, *Les médecins de l'Quest,* V. II, p 530; Doctors were very concerned with the problem in the 1840s: Weisz, *Ibid.*

45. Léonard and Sussman.

46. Dr. Lavarenne, "l'Encombrement médical," *Bul. des Syn méd. de France,* (April, 1900), p 906; Dr. Gouffier, "Le Malaise médical," *Bulletin Officiel des Sociétés médicales d'Arrondissement et du Conseil général des Sociétés du Département de la Seine* V. 4, N. VIII, (April 20, 1901), pp 202-204.

47. Brouardel, *La Profession médicale,* p 39.

48. Dr. Gouffier, "Le Malaise médical," *Bul. Off. des Soc. méd. d'Arron,* V. 4, N. Vii, (April 20, 1901),; Dr. A. Gassot, "l'Encombrement médical," *Bul. des Syn. méd de France,* (April, 1900), pp 904-906; Duchesne, "l'Encombrement médical. Moyen pratique d'y rémédier," *Ibid,* (Dec., 1899), p 859; "Le Péril médical," *Ibid,* (April, 1899), pp 763-765.

49. Dr. X, "De l'Encombrement médical," *Bul. des Syn. méd. de France,* (Feb. 1900), ppp 887-888.

50. 1870: Paris, Strasbourg, Montpellier; 1896: Faculties of Medicine: Paris, Montpellier, Nancy, Faculties of Medicine and Pharmacy: Bordeaux, Lille, Lyon, Toulouse.

51. After 1885, in addition to the baccalaureate in Latin and Greek, students could enter with a degree in Latin and living languages, Latin and Science, or French and Science. Another change which increased the numbr of students was a decision by the Paris faculty in 1884 to admit foreign sudents in an "open door" policy. Ostensibly these students were to return to practice in their own countries, however, apparently a substantial number of them stayed in the country.

52. *Ecoles en Plein Exercise* (four in 1896): Alger, Marseille, Nantes and Rennes. *Ecoles préparatoires de Médecine et de Pharmacy* (twelve in 1896): Amiens, Angers, Besançon, Caen, Clermont, Dijon, Grenoble, Limoges, Poitiers, Reims, Rouen, Tours.

53. *Gazette Hebd. des sciences médicales de Bordeaux*, V. 12, N. 34, (August 23, 1891, p 405.

54. Dr. Guionnet, "l'Encombrement médical,: *Bul. des Synd. méd. de France*, (August 1900), p 958; Dr. Maurice Lesieur, *Répértoire Officiel de la médecine et de la pharmacie française*, Paris, 1896. pp 9-20; Brouardel, *Ibid*, pp 17-18.

55. Martha L. Hildreth, "The Foundations of the Modern Medical System in France: Physician, Public Health Advocates and the Medical Legislation of 1892 and 1893," *Proceedings of the Western Society for French History*, 1980; Michel Boyer, "l'Encadrement médical dans l'Ardèche du XIX Siècle," *Revue du Vivarais*, V. 82, N. 653, (Jan., 1978), pp 16-31; Léonard, *Ibid.;* Sussman, *Ibid.* By practitioner, I include *docteurs* and *officiers de santé*.

56. See Chapter VI.

57. Hildreth, *Ibid.*

58. Maurice Agulhon, *La Vie Sociale en Provence intérieure au lendemain de la Révolution,* 1970.

59. Commune population of 10,000 was used as the criterion for urban versus rural; Dr. Lavarenne, "l'Encombrement médical," *Bul. des Syn. méd. de France,* (April, 1900) p 906.

60. Brouardel, *Ibid,* p 43.

61. See for example, *Gazette Hebd, des Sciences médicales de Bordeaux,* V. 13, N. 11, (Mars. 1892), p 132; Brouardel also wrote that he frequently received requests from local officials asking him to send them a doctor, *Ibid.,* p 44.

62. "Chronique Professionnelle," *Le Concours,* V. 9, N. 25, (June 18, 1887), pp 293.

63. Broardel, *La Profession médicale,* p 39, According to Brouardel the number of *médecins* in Paris increased from 1963 in 1893 to 2846 in 1900.

64. "Trop de médecins partout", *Le Concours,* V. 9, N. 31, (July 30, 1887), p 370.

65. *Ibid.;* Dr. Eugene Henriet, "Le Sage campagne menée par le Concours médical pour lutter contre l'Encombrement," *Bul. des Syn. méd. de France,* (May 1900) p 923.

66. *Ibid.* "l'Enquête sur l'Encombrement médical," *Le Concours,* V. 23, N. 9, pp 93-94.

67. "Un Docteur Qui Meurt de Faim," *Bul. Off. de l'Union des Syn. méd. de France,* (June 11, 1903)., pp 220-221; *Le Concours,* V. 1, N. 7, (Aug. 15, 1879).

68. *Société de protection des victimes du dévoir médical: Le Concours,* V. 14, N. 4, (Jan. 23, 1892), p 47.

69. "Chronique Professionnelle," *Le Concours,* V. 9, N. 25, (June 18, 1887), pp 293.

70. see for example: *Le Courrier médical et la Réforme médicale* (hereinafter Le Courrier médical), V. 41, N. 5, (Jan 31, 1891), p 49: *Lyon Médical,* N. 19, (May 7, 1893), p 33; *Gazette médicale de Liège,* V. 5, N. 30, (April 7, 1893) p 360.

71. Dr J. Bach, "Clients Refractaires," *La Fédération médicale,* N. 7, (Feb. 1897), pp 4-8.

72. Brouardel, *La Résponsabilité médicale,* Paris, 1898, p 8.

73. Bach, *Ibid.*

74. Dr Aymard, "Les premiers effets de l'Encombrement," *Bul. des Syn. méd. de France,* (May, 1901) pp 1038-1039.

75. Annon., "Statistique médicale de la France," *Journal de la Société de statistique de Paris,* V. 25 (1884), pp 114-5.

76. Dr. Aymard, *Ibid.*

77. Dr. Greletty, "Le mal et le bien qu'on a dit des médecins," *Le Concours,* V. 13, N. 32, (August 9, 1891), p 374-75; N. 22, (August 15, 1891), pp 386-387; Greletty even published a list of popular humorous anecdotes, which made fun at the expense of doctors. His purpose was

not to amuse but to warn doctors that they must work to change their public image.

78. Dr. Greletty, "Apologie du médecin de campagne," *Le Concours,* V. 13, N. 23, (June 6, 1891), p 266.

79. Brouardel, *La Profession médicale.*

80. Hoarce Bianchon, (pseud. for Maurice de Fleury), *Nos Grandes Médecins d'Aujourd'hui,* 1891.

81. *Le Concours,* V. 12, N. 40, (Oct. 4, 1890), pp 467-77.

82. *Bul. Off. de l'Union des Syn. méd. de France,* N. 5, (March 1902), p 98.

83. Cézilly, "Médecine et médecins," *Le Concours,* V. 9, N. 33, (August 13, 1887), pp 802-804.

84. "Une médiation à offrir," *Bul. des Syn méd. de France,* (March 1900).

85. "Les syndicats médicaux," *Gazette médicale de Lîège,*" V. r, N. 2, (Oct. 8, 1891).

86. *Ibid.*

87. Dr. E. Cacaille, "Nécessité d'Organiser la lutte contre les sociétés cooperatives," *Bul. des Syn. méd. de Nord et de Pas-de-Calais,* N. 8, (August 1901), pp 116-17); Brouardel, *La Profession médicale,* pp 47-48.

88. Dr. Grasset, *Bul. des Soc. méd. d'Arrond.,* V. 3, N. XVIII, (Sept. 20, 1900), p 547-48.

89. *Ibid.; Bul. des Syn. méd. de Lille.* N. 14, (July 1900), pp 209-10.

90. *Bul. des Soc. méd. d'Aron.*, V. 3, N. XVIII, (Sept. 20, 1900), pp 548-9; *Bul. des Syn. méd. de Lille,* N. 14, (July 1900), pp 209-10.

91. Cézilly, "Un médecin par commune!," *Le Concours,* V. 9, N. 25, (June 18, 1887), pp 293-94.

92. *Le Concours* V. 13, N. 42, (Oct. 17, 1891), p 501; "Syndicat des Vosges, l'Exercise des sages-femmes," *Le Concours,* V. 13, N. 18, (May 2, 1891), p 214; "La Tuberculose et les Charlatans," *Gazette Hebd. des Sciences médicales de Bordeaux,* V. 12, N. 25, (June 21, 1891), p 299.

93. "Un Singulier médecin," *Le Concours,* V. 10, N. 26, (June 30, 1888), pp 311-12.

94. *Bul Off. de l'Union des Syn. méd. de France,* N. 14, (July 20, 1903) pp 294-95.

95. Martin S. Pernick, "Medical Professionalism," James G. Burrom, "Organized Medicine," *Encyclopedia of Bioethics,* 1978, pp 1028-1030; Rodney Cole, *The Sociology of Medicine* 1978, pp 197-229.

96. Freidson, *Ibid.,* p 20-21; The medicine and practices of nineteenth century doctors was known as "heroic medicine" in the United States. Sarah Stage suggests that the popularity of patent medicines in the nineteenth century was a result of people seeking alternative to the treatments they received from doctors: Stage, *Female Complaints. Lydia Pinkham and the Business of Women's Medicine* 1979.

97. Pierre Guillaume, "Malades, médecine et médecins à Bordeaux au XIX Siècle," *Annales de Bretagne*, V. 86, N. 2, pp 291-300; *Gazette du Village*, V. 2, N. 5, (Feb. 2, 1890). p 56; *Le Courrier médical* recommended an infusion of rose petels as cure for diarrhea, which was thought to work because it functioned as an "antispectic" and "fermenticide:" *Le Courrier médical*, V. 41, N. 12, (Mars. 21, 1891), p 122.

98. Grellety, *Ibid.*

99. "Traitement de l'Hemorragie cérébrale," *Le Concours*, V. 1, N. 6, (Aug. 9, 1879), p 71; the recommended treatment was bleeding from a vein in the arm of 180 to 200 grams of blood.

100. *Le Concours*, V. 14, N. 9, (Feb. 27, 1892), p 105.

101. *Le Courrier médical*, V. 42, N. 49, (Dec. 3, 1892), p 419.

102. *Gazette Hebd. des Sciences médicales de Bordeaux*, V. 12, N. 22, (May 31, 1891), p 353; *Le Concours*, V. 1, N. 3, (July 19, 1879), p 36; in the 1890s there was a Société française d'éléctrotherapie in existence and a *Revue internationale d'éléctrotherapie*.

103. *Gazette médicale de Liège*, V. 5, N. 46, (Aug. 17, 1893), p 547. The electric bath consisted in placing the patient in a warm salt bath. A positive pole of an electric generator ("volta-faradique de Gaiffe, modèle moyen), was placed in the bath water. The negative pole was injected in a basin of water in which the patient's hand was immersed. The formerly comatose patient was revived!.

104. *Le Concours*, V. 14, N. 45, (Nov. 5, 1892), p 536.

105. "Les Laveurs Vagino-Uterins, Dit Vide-Bouteilles," *Gazette Hebd. des Sciences médicales de Bordeaux,* V. 13, N. 10, (Mar 6, 1892); *Le Courrier médical,* V. 41, N. 4, (Jan 24, 1891), p 40; "Les dangers due lavage de l'estomac," *Le Courrier médical,* V. 42, N. 49, (Dec. 3, 1892), p 419.

106. Freidson, pp 169-179.

107. Larson, *Ibid.*

108. Dr. F. Ranse, "Le médecin et la médecine de nos jours," *Gazette médicale de Paris.,* Series 7, V. VI, N. 14, (April 6, 1889), p 165.

109. Clement-Petit, *Ibid.*

110. Gouffier, "le malaise médical," *Bul. des Soc. méd. d'Arron.* V. 4, N. VIII, (April 20, 1901), pp 202-206; Bach, *Ibid;* Dr. J. Brasseur, "Les Syndicats professionnels," *Gazette médicale de Liège,* V. 5, N. 4, (Oct. 27, 1892), pp 36-27; Brouardel, *La Profession médicale,* pp 38-39, Brouardel arrived at the conclusion that there were fewer patients based on his observation that there were fewer deaths; an illustration of how poorly health and medical statistics were understood at the time.

111. Drs. Cayla and Malbec, "Conseil général des Sociétés d'Arrondissement," *Bul. des Soc. méd d'Arron,* (V. 4, N. XXI, (Nov. 5, 1901), pp 483-489.

112. Dr. Clement-Petit, *Ibid.*

113. Drs. Cayla and Malbec, "Conseil général des Sociétés d'Arrondissement," *Bul. des Soc. méd d'Arron,* (v. 5, N. XXI, (Nov. 5, 1901), pp 483-489.

114. Dr. Thierry, "Considerations sur les causes de la crise médicale actuelle," *Bul des Soc. méd. d'Arron.,* V. 3, N. VII, (April 5, 1900), p 268; Clement-Petit, *Ibid.,* Gouffier, *Ibid.*

115. *Gazette hebd. des Sciences médicales de Bordeaux,* V. 12, N. 8, (Feb. 22, 1891), p 94; *Gazette médicale de Paris,* Series 7, V. VIII, N. 13, (Mar. 28, 1891), pp 152-53; V. Vii, N. 39, (Sept. 23, 1886).

116. Dr. Clement-Petit, "Réponse à Dr. Gouffier," *Bul. Off. des Soc. méd. d'Arron.,* V. 4, N. VII, (April 20, 1901), pp 204-212; "l'Exploitation de l'Assistance publique par les malades aises," *Bul. de l'Union des Syn. méd. de France,* (June 1893), p 801-802. The Pasteur Institute was founded in Paris in 1885, thus beginning a wave of clinic and dispensary creation in the principle cities of the nation. Clement-Petit noted that the clinic newly founded in his neighborhood charged its patients only 20 centimes, and that only to those patients who could afford to pay.

117. Dr. Lande, "Les payantes dans les hôpitaux," *Ibid;* "Les Malades aises dans les Hôpitaux," *La Fédération médicale,* N. 22 (May, 1898), pp 6-8.

118. Dr. Quercy, *Ibid; Le Concours,* V. 14, N. 34, N. 17, (April 23, 1892), p 194; v. 15, N. 34, (Aug. 20, 1892), p 405; V. 15, N. 37, (Sept. 16, 1893), p 444; *Bul. de l'Union des Syn. méd. de France,* (June 1893), pp 801-02; (June 1901), p 1082.

119. Dr. Quercy, *La France médicale,* V. 39, N. 18, (April 19, 1892).

120. Génésteix, *Ibid.*

121. Cézilly "Les syndicats médicaux à Paris," *Le Concours,* V. 14, N. 12, (Mar. 19, 1892), pp 140-43.

122. See chapter Five.

123. Michel Foucault, *The Birth of the Clinic,* 1972.

124. Dr. C... "l'Abus de l'Hôpital et des Soins gratuits," *Bul. des Syn. méd. de France,* (May, 1900), pp 926-927.

125. Dr. Duchesne, "Quelques rémarques sur la crise médicale," *Bul. des Syn. méd. de France* (Oct. 1900); Duchesne said he was speaking for Jeanne, Gassot, and Boyer of the Union governing board.

126. Brouardel, *La Profession médicale,* pp 45-47.

127. Broardel, *Ibid.*

128. M. Dromain, *Bul. Off. des Soc. méd. d'Arron.,* V. 4, N. IV, Feb. 20, 1901; Dr. J. Bach, "Pauvres médecins de la beau pays de France," *La Féderation médicale,* N. 4, (Nov. 1896), p 7; Dr. Le Maguet, *Le Concours,* V. 14, N. 15, (April 16, 1892), p 191.

129. Dr. F. Boe, "Les Concours médicaux et les Juifs," *Bul. des Soc. méd. d'Arron.,* V. 3, N. xiii, (July 5, 1900), p 455.

130. *Le Concours,* V. 23, N. 9, (Mar. 2, 1901) pp 93-94.

CHAPTER II
THE NATIONAL PUBLIC HEALTH BUREAUCRACY AND THE
BACTERIOLOGICAL REVOLUTION

French hygienists of the late nineteenth century were in a better position than ever to make an impact on the nation's health. For the first time, political concerns and social ideology were favorable to legislation which would intervene into areas formerly left to the family and local society. In addition, hygienists possessed a scientific theory which could be experimentally validated and which offered specific solutions to disease. And yet, in spite of the overwhelmingly favorable climate, particularistic concerns created substantial barriers to public health activity. One of these barriers came from Senators anxious to protect property rights. Another barrier came from doctors anxious to protect their own most valuable property, their private practice.

For decades the French National Public Health Committee, the Comité consultatif d'Hygiène publique (C.C.H.P.), was a mostly ignored stepchild of the Ministry of Commerce and Agriculture. However, the events of the 1880s and early 1890s brought glamour and prestige to the C.C.H.P. and more importantly brought it the attention of the government. The discoveries of the bacteriological revolution provided the C.C.H.P. with rather straightforward and relatively simple answers to the two most serious contagious diseases which ravaged France in this period, cholera and typhoid. Moreover, the committee members produced statistical studies which proved the likelihood of positive results from the measures they recommended. The C.C.H.P. also benefited from the populationist anxiety and solidarist orientation of the government. Several prominent progressive legislators sat on the committee and promoted its programs in the Chamber and Senate. In 1888, indicating its new importance, the committee was transferred from the Ministry of Agriculture and put in the Ministry of Interior under the directorship of the noted scientist, bureacrat and partisan of solidarist ideology, Henri Monod.

The history of the C.C.H.P. and is predecessor, the *Conseil supérieur de la Santé* was closely linked to the ongoing debates over the etiology of disease in the nineteenth century. For centuries contagion theory had risen and fallen in popularity, competing with several other conflicting theories of the origins of diseases. [1] Contagion reached perhaps its lowest level of repute in the mid nineteenth century at precisely the same time that Louis Pasteur and Robert Koch were performing the experiments which would eventually lead to the establishment of germ theory. [2] The most popular theory of disease at this time was the old theory of miasma, espoused by Galen, questioned in the Middle Ages and popular in subsequent centuries. [3] According to the miasma theory, disease was caused by the inhalation of bad air, that is, air polluted by sources such as smelly swamps and putrefying animal matter. In miasma theory metereological conditions were seen as important because air pressure, humidity, and wind all played a role in concentrating or dispersing air. According to the theory, certain locales were inherently unhealthy because of the climate, topography or the presence of certain industries. [4] Long before the work of Pasteur and Koch, scientists had questioned miasma and speculated on the role of microbes in diseases such as diphtheria, cholera, smallpox, and puerperal (childbed) fever. In the mid nineteenth century, however, miasma was again in vogue, contagion theory was derided, and the scientists who espoused contagion saw their reputations badly abused. [5]

The *Conseil supérieur de la santé,* the central French Public Health Committee from 1822 to 1848, was a backwater of contagionism while the dominant medical and public opinion was anti-contagionist. The *Conseil supérieur* was founded in 1822 in response to the yellow fever epidemic which threatened France from Spain in that year. [6] During the subsequent decades, the activities of the council stagnated, in part due to the disinterest of the Restoration and July Monarchy in public health matters, and in part to the medical controversies between contagionists and anti-contagionists. The *Conseil supérieur's* efforts to stop yellow fever and cholera epidemics by shutting off frontiers to immigration, travel and trade were completely ineffectual and worked to discredit both the council and contagion theory. [7] During the 1830s and 1840s, the council continued to exist but with no funds and no clear functions, its role was simply advisory. In spite of the absence of an effective central public health bureaucracy, the public health movement was far from inactive in France in the first half of the nineteenth century, as Ann F. La Berge has clearly demonstrated. [8] Hygienists made some progress in effecting reform, mostly in Paris. However, although this movement included numerous hard-working and dedicated scientists, engineers, and doctors it made little headway as far as national legislation was concerned.

Under the dominant miasmatic theory, the kinds of reforms necessary to prevent disease were vast and daunting. According to the miasmatic public health movement, disease had to be countered through a complete cleanup of the environment incuding shops, streets, factories and homes. Disease could only be prevented by providing adequate and sanitary living, working and breathing space for all citizens. George Rose and Erwin Ackerknecht have pointed out that this theory was in keeping with the liberal temperment of the time, whereas the implications of contagion theory ran counter to it. [9]

Miasmatic public health called for extensive social reform to equalize the living conditions of the classes. The great hygienist and statistician, Louis-René Villermé, pointed out that the basic cause of miasmas was economic: poverty created crowded and unhealthy conditions. [10] This theory suited both fatalists and activists. The fatalists believed that since poverty was unavoidable so was disease. The liberal reformers worked to implement a variety of programs to improve working class life, although only socialists carried Villermé's insights to their logical conclusion. But it was the fatalists who generally triumphed.

Contagion theory, on the other hand, implied a degree of interference in people's lives which nineteenth century liberal ideology found untenable. Since the paths of contagion were unknown, all substances were subject. Thus contagionists often called for restrictions on all trade and travel during epidemics. As Rosen and Ackerknecht have indicated, the measures taken against smallpox and yellow fever in the early part of the century were seen as intolerable by commercial interests. In the late nineteenth century, however, social and medical ideology began to change.

The Second Republic made a new commitment to public health and founded the C.C.H.P. in August 1848. The C.C.H.P. was re-created in the same form under Presidential decree in February, 1850. The C.C.H.P. was to replace the inactive *Conseil supérieur de la santé* and was likewise placed under the Ministry of Agriculture and Commerce. [11] In its early years, the C.C.H.P. operated mainly as a forum for discussion and communication between the numerous scientists, physicians and engineers with interests and functions pertaining to health issues. The primary subjects of discussion were unsafe and unhealthy housing and working conditions and adulterated food and drink. [12] The committee's main goal in this time was to create a national network of public health councils, extending down to the departmental and arrondissement levels, which would connect the entire nation with the top expertise on public health. It was hoped that these local councils would investigate cases of unhealthy work, living and commercial conditions as well as comercial fraud. Further, the

C.C.H.P. hoped that these local councils would provide information and statistics back to the central authority on epidemics and endemic disease, so that for the first time the central government would have a reliable and comprehensive picture of health conditions. However, these efforts, although strongly backed by the government, met with frustration after frustration, as local authorities simply refused to cooperate. In spite of repeated efforts by the C.C.H.P. and the Ministry of Agriculture, by 1861 only about one-quarter of the departments had actively functioning departmental health councils. [13] Over the next two decades, however, the C.C.H.P. made some progress in creating departmental councils, so that by 1882 about three-quarters of all departments had functioning public health councils. In addition, there were about 185 arrondissement councils by 1884. [14] Some of these councils even had inspectors attached to them and were regularly hearing reports on cases of unhealthy conditions. However, most of the councils were only used as advisory bodies to the prefects.

In the 1870s and 1880s, these departmental and arrondissement councils compiled hundreds of reports on unhealthy conditions in workplaces, schools, cemeteries, roads, water supplies, drains, dumps, slaughterhouses, factories, and homes. However, as the members of the C.C.H.P. often noted, it was one thing to identify health problems and quite another thing to get local officials to do anything about them. In compiling the record of the work of the local health councils, Dr. Vallin of the C.C.H.P. noted that it seemed as if local officials only got concerned about a health problem if it clearly threatened commercial nterests. [15]

Because of the effects of miasmatic theory, public health was seen
s a concept relevant principally to industrial, urban environments. Most
prefects, subprefects and departmental councilors could not see the util-
ty of it outside of the cities. Disease was thought to be caused by bad
air resulting from the concentration of agents of putrification; therefore,
areas where people, food and sewage were dispersed and where the air
generally smelled and felt fresh, were thought to be healthy and in no
need of the attention of public authorities. Disease occurring in rural
areas were usually explained by the visit of the victims to some oter
unhealthy area, or to some temporary and coincidental miasmatic
phenomenon. [16]

The only significant achievement of the C.C.H.P. in its early years
was the passing of the 1858 law on dangerous lodgings. The law was
ntended to combat the unhealthy atmosphere of many working class
districts in the cities. However, this law was ineffectual because the
C.C.H.P. and the local health councils had no ability to levy sanctions.

Frustrated by the lack of cooperation on the part of local officials,
he C.C.H.P. of the Third Republic argued that a law needed to be
passed which would force the local governments to take responsibility
n areas of public health and give the C.C.H.P. the authority to determine what kind of measures should be taken. However, in the 1870s
and 1880s the upper echelons of the bureaucracy and the government
seemed to believe that such a measure was too drastic. The Ministeries

of Interior and Agriculture encouraged the C.C.H.P.'s efforts to pressure local officials to create and use health councils, but refused to become involved in a public health law.

In 1884, in the midst of a terrible cholera epidemic, the government passed a law which enabled mayors to take drastic and extensive actions to stop the spread of the disease and procure treatment for victims. However, the law only gave the mayors the prerogative to take anti-epidemic measures, not the responsibility to do so. Moreover, municipal councils were not required to vote funds to support this activity, and in most communes the law had little effect. Henri Monod and members of the C.C.H.P. saw this law as a step backward in public health beacuse it implied that local officials, not the C.C.H.P., were the primary public health agents. At the same time the law did not require the locals to take any actions. [17] It was not until Henri Monod took over the direction of public health that the Ministry of the Interior committed itself to a national public health law. [18]

The C.C.H.P.'s lack of success before the 1890s can be attributed in part to the confusion over contagion and miasma. It was in the seventies that Pasteur's theories were being hotly debated at the Academy of Medicine. His reception was so hostile that Pasteur gave up going to the Academy of Medicine and confined his reports to the more receptive Academy of Science. Finally Pasteur's ideas won popularity after his successful us of the Anthrax anti-toxin in 1881 and the rabies vaccine in 1885. In Germany, Robert Koch was also making major breakthroughs. In 1882 he identified the cause of tuberculosis and in the same year his student, Carl Klebs, identified the diphtheria bacillus. In 1884 Koch identified the cholera bacterium. [19] However, the work of Koch and Pasteur and their students left many questions unanswered, such as what microbes were, where they congregated and how they were transmitted. The greatest question revolved around the controversy over spontaneous generation. This old theory in effect combined contagion and miasma by holding that certain atmospheric conditions caused the spontaneous generation of microbes or grains which in turn caused disease. [20] The theory thus put the emphasis back on miasmas as the basic cause of disease. Thus, although Pasteur's experiments would seem to have effectively refuted this theory by the 1870s, it was still widely believed.

Whereas their predecessors on the *Conseil supérieur* had been staunchly pro-contagionist, many members of the C.C.H.P. were simply very confused in the 1870s and 1880s. Members frequently discussed "germs" and "miasmas" as if they were really just the same phenomenon. In 1880, in a report on the most serious disease of children, three of the council's most prestigious scientists encouraged isolation of victims stricken with these diseases because of the danger of "transmission of miasmas." [21] In the 1880s, at the faculties of medicine in Paris and Bordeaux, the hygiene courses of doctors Bouchardat, Proust, and Layet focused on a wide variety of subjects including magnetism, humidity, electricity, light, atmospheric pressure, climate, ethnology, and temperaments as well as "grains" and "germs." Thus the educated elites of medical education were beginning to accept the idea of germs and contagion but tended to weld this to miasmatic theory. Swamps, drains, cisterns, wells, dumps, and sewage were studied as sources of contamination, but it was not clear whether the source of contamination was in air, matter or water. While recognizing the need for isolation and disinfection, most hygienists were still very puzzled over how contagion took place and what sorts of living organisms (germs) or inorganic substances (grains) were involved. In addition to germs and miasmas, the hygiene courses of Bouchardat, Proust and Layet also discussed the popular concern with the role of inherited traits and personality characteristics which were held responsible for a number of diseases including syphilis, tuberculosis, alcoholism and nervous disorders. *Hygiène,* then, was a complex and many-faceted issue and hygienists had no clear and easy answers to give as to what public health measures had to be taken to stop the course of the major diseases.

The confusion over miasma and germ theory began to be resolved as new members entered the C.C.H.P. between 1884 and 1889 from the *Société de médecine publique et d' hygiène profesionnelle.* Most important of these was Paul Brouardel, who was made president of the C.C.H.P. in 1884, at which time he was on his way to becoming the most important medical bureaucrat in the nation. Brouardel remained president of the C.C.H.P. until 1903. Another important member of both the society and the C.C.H.P. was Dr. André Jusin (A.J.) Martin, who became an official member of the C.C.H.P. in 1889. [22] Martin was the secretary of the *Société de Médecine publique de d'Hygiène professionnelle,* secretary of the C.S.A.P. after 1889, chief health inspector for the city of Paris and the architect of the 1902 Public Health Law. Brouardel and Martin were followers of Pasteur and although Pasteur himself was a member of the C.C.H.P. from 1881 until his death in 1895, his advanced age and poor health left Brouardel and Martin as leaders of Pasteurian public health on the C.C.H.P. Other important new members of the C.C.H.P. in this period who were also members of the *Société de Médecine publique et d'hygiène profession-nelle* included Drs. Jacques Bertillon, Desirè-Magloire Bourneville, Lèon Colin, Andrè-Victor Cornil, Du Mesnil, Henri Napias, Emile Roux and Adrien Proust. Bertillon was the chief of the statistic bureau of the City of Paris, a bureau which had been created by his father, Louis Adolphe Bertillon. The Bertillons and the *Société de la statistique de Paris* were responsible for bringing to light the declining French population statistics which so alarmed the upper classes of French society in the late nineteenth and early twentieth centuries. Bourneville was also a deputy and Cornil a Senator; Colin and Du Mesnil were chiefs of the national asylum at Vincennes. Colin was later Minister of War, and president of the Academy of Médicine. Napias, who co-authored a number of hygiene works with Martin, was the chief inspector of assistance services for the National Public Assistance Council (C.S.A.P.). Roux was Pasteur's long-time collaborator and a member of both the Academies of Medicine and Science. He was also an under-director of the newly created Pasteur Institute. Finally, Proust was a prestigous medical bureaucrat who was a member of the Academy of Medicine, professor of hygiene at the Paris Faculty and chief inspector of national sanitary services, and perhaps most importantly, the father of Marcel Proust.

The *Société de Médecine publique et d'hygiène professionnelle* was founded in 1877 to promote public health legislation in France. Most of the members were disciples of Pasteur. The society was very critical of France's poor record in health legislation as compared to England, Germany and Belgium. Its initial goals were to centralize all public health authority under one ministry and see the passage of a law making smallpox vaccination mandatory for all citizens. The society also worked to establish more urban hygiene bureaus and laboratories and to gather more precise health statistics. In the face of a terrible typhoid epidemic in Paris in 1882, members of the society began to agitate for the creation of a unified and centralized public health authority in France. They publicized their ideas in the forum of the Academy of Medicine and the pages of the hygiene journals as well as in the popular press. [23] In the 1880s, the goals and programs of the society became those of the C.C.H.P. Under the leadership of Brouardel, Martin and Jacques Bertillon, the C.C.H.P. was dedicated to the precise determination of the agents and means of contagion and their eradication, as well as to the comprehensive and accurate compilation of disease and death statistics.

1889 was an important year for the C.C.H.P. A microbiological laboratory was established and France's first epidemiological service was organized. These services began the long project of examining the water supplies of French cities. Also in 1889, the C.C.H.P. was put under the authority of Minister of the Interior, Léon Bourgeois and his under-director, Henri Monod. Bourgeois's and Brouardel's formal addresses to the C.C.H.P. at the beginning of that year illustrate the social ideas which underlay the C.C.H.P.'s subsequent rise to prominence in the 1890s. Brouardel warned that France's population was growing very slowly, while that of neighboring nations had doubled in forty or fifty years. The government, he pointed out, could do nothing about the birth rate, but it sould made an impact on mortality. Brouardel went on to state that thanks to recent discoveries, hygienists were beginning to understand the causes of typhoid, cholera and dysentery and how to combat them. Thus, Brouardel urged the legislature to support the legislative goals and hygiene programs of the C.C.H.P.

Léon Bourgeois likewise noted the slow growth of the French population over the last century. Now was the time, he said, to organize a truly effective health bureaucracy to do something about the mortality rates from contagious disease. According to Bourgeois, to fight such diseases was "to take on a battle for democracy and fraternal society." It was, he said, the work of the strong of the nation to aid the weak. Bourgeois said he counted on Monod and Brouardel to put Pasteur's discoveries into action. [24] Bourgeois clearly recognized that potential conflict existed between solidarist and hygienists on one hand and the defenders of a certain concept of individual liberty on the other. His comments are worth quoting at length for they show how the solidarist medical legislation of the period represented the beginnings of state interventionist social ideology in France.

Bourgeois noted that the formation of a centralized direction for public health,

> "...should not worry the defenders of individual liberty...When public powers take measures to safeguard the health of the population, two conditions must be rigorously met. The scientific validity of the measures prescribed must be beyond all serious challenge. The population cannot in any case serve as the experimental grounds for scientific theories. In matters of hygiene, the state does not have the right to interfere in the progress of science. It is up to science to speak for itself and to execute its own experiments without harming the liberty of citizens.
>
> In addition, the measures prescribed by public health authorities should not interfere with individual liberty any more than necessary for the preservation of life and health. ...Personal hygiene, of course, is of incontestable benefit for the individual but it cannot be imposed on him... However, when it is no longer just a question of the harm that an individual does to himself, but of the harm which he does to others; when it is a question of defending the health of his neighbors, the renters of his building, the population of a commune or city, the children in our schools, and the soldiers of our army, menaced by a source of contagion, the extent of public powers is governed by the right to protect each of the lives menaced, and at the same time, the right of existence makes the right to protect into a duty to act.
>
> [The powers of public health] will conform to the principles of our democratic republic: because the powers benefit the weak, the little people, and the unfortunate, and because they are aimed at conserving and expanding human capital, the smallest parcel of which cannot be lost without harming the security of

the nation and the glory of the country. They embody the demand of patriotism." [25]

As Bourgeois noted, the C.C.H.P. had to prove the efficacy of its anti-contagion measures in order to call for government action. The typhoid and cholera epidemics which ravaged France in the 1880s and 1890s gave the C.C.H.P. the opportunity it needed to do so. The epidemics greatly alarmed populationist anxieties. But more importantly, these epidemics were meticulously studied by members of the C.C.H.P. and gradually yielded evidence that pointed to the critical role of water supply in the etiology of the diseases.

In the years 1882-1883 and 1886-1889 typhoid was a major cause of death. Members of the C.C.H.P. noted that typhoid was a severe and endemic health problem in France which had not been given nearly the attention it deserved. Cholera was the most feared disease of the 1880s and 1890s because of its high mortality rate (seventy to eighty per cent). Typhoid, however, actually caused more deaths overall. [26] Hygientists noted that in the period 1872 through 1889, incidents of typhoid in France had greatly increased, at the very same time that the disease was becoming less frequent in Germany and Austria. [27] Statistics reported for 195 of the largest French cities showd 4,682 deaths from typhoid in 1886, or 5.45 for every 10,000 inhabitants; there were 5,879 in 1887, or 6.85 for 10,000 inhabitants; and 4,720 in 1888, or 5.5 for 10,000 inhabitants. In the 195 cities for which statistics were reported in the period 1886-1888, typhoid was the single biggest killer among all infectious diseases, although measles was a close second. [28]

Typhoid caused great social disruption as witnessed by an epidemic in Clermont-Ferrand in the fall and winter of 1886; 8,000 people left town when the cases of typhoid reached a rate of over 200 per day. [29] In the army garrisons, where the most accurate disease statistics were kept, the incidents of typhoid were even more appalling. Between 1875 and 1888 among the 5,663,412 men who belonged to the Army of the Interior, there were 16,177 deaths from typhoid. [30] The scattered reports available on typhoid in rural areas indicates that rural Frenchmen were often as susceptible as their urban brothers and sisters. A study of the rural canton of Baccarat (Meurthe-et-Moselle) for the years 1856-1880 showed severe endemic typhoid. There were frequent cases of whole households of four to six persons victimized by the same epidemic with thirty per cent mortality. Communes of four to seven hundred inhabitants reported ten to twenty per cent of their population struck with the disease in some years. [31]

In the 1880s there was intense controversy among hygienists as to the way in which typhoid was transmitted. The studies of the Englishmen Murchisson and Budd, published in 1856 and 1862, found the source of typhoid to be in both water and air. In 1865 the Germans Buhl and Pettenkofr demonstrated the association of incidents of typhoid and low levels of subterranian water; however, they gave this phenomenon a miasmatic explanation. Buhl and Pettenkofr maintained that the agent which caused typhoid was in the soil, and was transferred to the surface by water pressure and released into the air. The respected French scientist, A. Durand-Claye, also subscribed to a miasmatic explanation. He made a detailed study of typhoid in Paris in 1883 and concluded that the disease was the result of an "ensemble of factors," including climate, water pressure, geology and contamination. [32] Likewise, Dr. Alison's lengthy study of rural typhoid insisted that bad air was the principal cause of the disease. [33] In the late 1880s, Brouardel and the French scientist, Auguste Adrien Ollivier, refuted the theories of Buhl and Pettenkofr and maintained the that the "principe morbifique" (casual principle) existed in the water itself. [34]

The C.C.H.P. began intense studies of the course of typhoid epidemics in order to settle the controversy. Between 1884 and 1892 the committee studies 455 projects to purify the drinking water of various urban communes and noted the relation between improvements and reductions in cases of typhoid. By 1888, the studies of Brouardel, André Chantemesse and Léon Henri Thoinot clearly implicated contaminated drinking water as the critical factor. Even so, Brouardel himself was reluctant to dismiss other sources of transmission and maintained as late as 1887 that the disease could be transmitted by clothes and air as well as by water and dirty hands. [35] In 1892, however, Brouardel, and therefore the official opinion of the C.C.H.P., diminished the role of air in the propagation of typhoid. The committee held that drinking water was the primary agent of transmission and that other means of transmission were secondary. Apparently the final proof was the success of Minister of War and hygienist, Léon Colin, in reducing the incidents of typhoid among the soldiers of the Army of the Interior by installing carbon filters in the water supplies of all garrisons. [36]

One of the barriers to the total destruction of miasmatic theory was the fact that laboratory techniques were in a primitive state. Therefore, although the bacillus of typhoid fever had been identifies by Carl Eberth in 1880, it could only occasionally be verified as present in suspect water in spite of the concerted detection efforts of Brouardel and his students. [37] The same applied to the detection of the cause of cholera. Although the bacillus had been identified by Koch, epidemiology researchers had difficulty establishing its presence in all outbreaks of the disease. As with typhoid, the popular theory as to the causes of cholera was that a "causal principle" existed which could attach itself to a number of different materials, but which was actually transmitted when it came into contact with air. [38] This theory was popular until the late 1880s when hygienists began to note that the same water projects which reduced the incidents of typhoid also resulted in less cholera. [39]

Major breakthroughs in cholera etiology were made in 1891 and 1892, when several investigators associated with the C.C.H.P. undertook studies which clearly demonstrated the critical role of water. Cholera was a terrifying phenomenon in the nineteenth century. The epidemic of 1884-86 took over 12,000 lives in France. [40] In 1891 measures prescribed by the C.C.H.P. made significant steps in stopping the spread of a cholera epidemic in Le Havre. Residents were advised to drink only boiled or bottled water, cholera victims were isolated in a special hospital pavilion, and the clothing and personal effects of the victims and their families were thoroughly disinfected. Hospital attendants were told to carefully dispose of the body wastes of their cholera patients and to disinfect and boil all articles coming into contact with them. Families who refused to take their cholera victims to the hospitals were told to do likewise. These measures seem to have stopped the Havre epidemic before it caused more than a few hundred cases and prevented the epidemic from spreading to the rest of the nation. However, in the following year a severe epidemic broke out in the department of the Seine and shortly thereafter throughout the nation.

The 1892 epidemic saw another important breakthrough in the identification of the etiology of cholera. Drs. Thoinot and Jean Baptiste Fernand Dubief, working as health inspectors for the Department of the Seine, clearly traced the origins of the outbreak in the Paris basin to the waters of the Seine and thereby proved the crucial role of drinking water in the spread of the disease. The first cases of the disease had occurred at the *Maison départementale* (departmental home for the aged and incompetent) at Nanterre and led the public to the belief, as miasmatic theory would imply, that this was a location of a bad miasma which was the source of the epidemic. [41] Several factors allowed the investigators to study closely the path of contamination, however, and to eliminate hypotheses which pointed to factors other than water. The *Maison départmentale* had been built since the cholera epidemic of 1884 and therefore could not be seen as a "foyer d'épidémie," a place where conditions were such that causal agents of cholera had remained present but dormant since the last epidemic. Also, the employees of the *maison* kept track of the comings and goings of the residents and visitors. Therefore the investigators could eliminate the hypothesis that the disease had been brought into the *maison* by an individual because no foreign visitors or new residents had entered for several weeks prior to the outbreak. Moreover, cholera was not known to be present anywhere in Europe prior to the outbreak in the Paris basin in 1892. Some of the *maison* residents were involved in the sorting of old clothes, but the investigators determined that they had not come into contact with shipments of discarded clothes from soldiers stationed in the far east. Therefore the investigators concluded that the epidemic had not originated in the *maison*, neither had it been brought there through the agency of a person or object. However, they concluded that because of the age, poor health, and close living conditions of the residents, the *maison* constituted an environment were an epidemic, once begun, would spread with unusual rapidity and deadliness. [42]

The question remained, how did the cholera epidemic at Nanterre begin? Dubief and Thoinot noted that the first three pensioners who came down with the disease at Nanterre were in the habit of going to drink daily in nearby communes, Corbevoie and Puteaux, where all drinking water came from the Seine. Within ten days after the first of these three pensioners came down with the disease, cases were reported at both these communes among people who had had no contact with the *maison* or any of its residents. Shortly thereafter a wide number of scattered cases of cholera occurred in several suburban communes aroung Paris all of which got their water supply from the same three pumping stations on the Seine. The investigators concluded that although they could not establish how the causal agent got into the water of the Seine, they could clearly pinpoint the water in that river as the source of contamination. [43]

For the first time the hygienists had overwhelming evidence that water was the primary agent of contamination. They also concluded that secondary transmission occurred in families and institutions where the members lived in a close and unclean environment and therefore came into contact with the body wastes of the cholera victims. Before the 1892 epidemic, investigators had noted that middle class and wealthy families were able to avoid cholera and typhoid by boiling all their water supplies and drinking bottled water, but poor families tended to spread the disease among themselves in spite of the same precautions. Also, by keeping track of the occupations of cholera victims in Paris in 1892, the scientists discoverd that there was a high incidence of the disease among occupational groups which were in frequent contact with water and raw food. [44]

These investigations had a crucial effect on public health legislation. Miasmas were clearly discredited in cholera and typhoid. Further, hygienists could point to one major source of transmission, drinking water. Thus some relatively simple measures could be taken by government authorities to eliminate these diseases. They no longer had to transform the whole environment, only to purify the water supply. The contrast between the C.C.H.P. recommendations at the time of the 1884 cholera epidemic and the 1892 epidemic illustrate this point. In 1884 the C.C.H.P. had recommended a comprehensive clean up of all homes and shops, streets, and gutters, and the closing of some butchers, stock yards, and wholesale food markets. Naturally many officials had balked at such stringent measures. In 1892, however, they recommended much simpler measures including isolation of the victim, attending to the cleanliness of his immediate environment and the use of boiled and bottled water. [45]

The cholera and typhoid epidemics of the period 1884-92 had other effects as well. It was not a mere coincidence that legislators passed a medical bill in 1892 and another in 1893. Deputies, Senators and bureaucrats were very alarmed by the ever lower birth rate and the consistently high moratlity rate of the French population. In the late 1880s, statistics showed an increasingly narrow margin of births over deaths, and Bertillon and Brouardel predicted that in the early 1890s the annual number of deaths would exceed the number of births. The typhoid and cholera epidemics of the period seemed to make true the dire warnings about the impending depopulation of France. Gerard Jacquemet called these epidemics and the accompanying population anxieties, the new "Great Fear." [46] However, it proved to be much easier to pass a law on the practice of medicine (1892) and a medical assistance law (1893) than a public health act. A public health act was drafted by the C.C.H.P. and passed by the Chamber of Deputies in 1893 in the middle of the cholera epidemic, but it did not make it through the Senate. It was nearly another decade before France passed a public health act. Much of the difficulty had to do with the reluctance of private doctors and conservative Senators to submit to the kind of interference and regulation that a public health authority implied. Another difficulty was convincing private physicians and the general public of the validity of the C.C.H.P.'s theories on the role of water in typhoid and cholera.

The C.C.H.P. found that local doctors were reluctant to accept the role of drinking water in the transmission of disease. In the case of the Clermont-Ferrand epidemic, Chantemesse and Brouardel had example after example pointing to the role of the city water, including cases where in the same household individuals who had drunk bottled or boiled water had been spared while others had succumbed. However, the majority of local doctors refused to believe that drinking water could cause the disease and clung to a miasmatic theory that bad air emanating from generally unhealthy conditions and overcrowding was the cause. [47] Brouardel also noted that municipal officials and the public in general were unwilling to accept the notion that impure water caused typhoid and cholera. Brouardel believed that city authorities feared the social and economic disruption that distrust of the water supply could cause. Also the average person could not understand how the water that he and his ancestors had drunk safely for years could become suddenly dangerous. [48]

Hygienists despaired at their inability to convince either the public or most private practitioners of the role which water played in contagious disease. The health council of the department of the Seine noted ironically that hundreds of Parisians escaped the bad miasmas of the city each week with a trip to supposedly healthy and picturesque Meudon. But at Meudon they drank the water of the Seine, badly contaminated because the village was downstream from Paris. There, the council members believed, many Parisians likely caught typhoid and other diseases. [49]

In the 1880s, the popular medical journals still expressed considerable scepticism toward germ theory. Physicians continued to confuse contagion theory and miasmatic concepts of disease. [50] In the early 1880s, Dr. A. Bechamp of Lille promoted a theory of "Microzymas" which rivaled Pasteur's microbe theory. Bechamp's theory espoused spontaneous generation in a combination of germ and miasma theory. [51] In the 1890s, doctors writing for a popular audience still implicated air temperature and atmosphere as the main causes of cholera and flu. [52] *Le Concours* gave a great deal of publicity to Koch's supposed development of an inoculation to treat tuberculosis, and when the technique subsequently proved useless, it became somewhat disenchanted, again, with germ theory. [53]

As the hygienists began to accept germ theory, they began to revive the once maligned theories of asepsis espoused by Joseph Lister in the 1860s. This was particularly true after the aseptic operation was performed in Germany in 1886. [54] It is difficult to know to what extent doctors in private practice were applying the principles of asepsis in the 1890s. Maurice de Fleury is probably a reliable witness on this issue because he was much admired by Cézilly and wrote generally in praise of the medical profession. [55] However, in 1890, Fleury had some critical comments to make about the inattention which doctors gave to contagion:

"Doctors themselves are not what they should be. Dr. Maurice Letulle, speaking of the role of practicians in the face of infectious disease, demonstrates that the doctor himself is doubtless an agent of transmission of illnesses. He cites numerous cases and don't we all know that the children of doctors themselves are frequently the victims of illnesses carried to them by their fathers?

...A practioner, whose name I will keep secret, absolutely refuses to admit the microbian doctrine. He supports his own theory, and recommends soiled dressings, as he puts it himself. One day he was permitted to perform an ovarotomy in these conditions; the woman died, naturally. This doctor is not a dishonest man; he does not kill for the pleasure of it..." [56]

Fleury found this inattention to asepsis to be inexcusable given what was widely known about microbe theory and contagion. To remedy the situation, he had some original recommendations. According to Fleury the public should take it upon itself to make sure that doctors were treating them under aseptic conditions. Fleury recommended that mothers observe the doctor when he visted to make sure that he washed his hands and face before and after his examination. Fleury pointed out that the washing of the face was necessary because osculation was performed with the doctor's ear next to the patient's body. According to Fleury, a mother should also inquire if the doctor had just come from a visit which involved a contagious disease, and if so insist upon ordering antiseptic solutions from the pharmacist for the doctor to wash with before his examination. The mother should also order fumigation and disinfection services for her home after a family illness, if the doctor neglected to do so. Finally, Fleury recommended that legislation be passed enforcing asepsis upon doctors. Cézilly, although he complimented Fleury as an "excellent medical writer," objected to his suggestions that the public become involved in monitoring the practices of doctors. He found Fleury's recommended procedures "Draconian"; they required too much time and trouble and would make the doctor "ridiculous." [57]

Outside of asepsis, there were initially few other technical breakthroughs that the average practitioner could implement. The other major improvements in health care involved clean water, safe food and adequate sewage disposal. All of these developments fell into the realm of public health application. There was considerable confusion in the mind of the public and doctors between private practitioners and the growing public health movement. In describing the profession at the end of the century Brouardel said that doctors were "hygienist" by definition. [58] This was simply not true. Contagion theory was not automatically accepted. Moreover, the syndicat movement opposed many of the reforms which the new bacteriological public health movement instigated.

In the 1880s the C.C.H.P. began to call for the enactment of five major health reforms. These included a more effective and centralized public health bureaucracy, water examination services, disinfection services, mandatory smallpox vaccination; dispensary services for contagious disease, and the requirement of declaration of cause of death and cases of contagious disease. Most of these reforms engendered the opposition of private physicians. The C.C.H.P. wanted to see the creation of a truly centralized and effective public health bureaucracy which would have the authority to cite and correct sources of disease. At the head of this bureaucracy would be the C.C.H.P. itself which would decree general measures and policy. The departments would be required to create and budget local councils which would be the arms of the C.C.H.P. These departmental councils would be headed by a director and joined by a professional inspection service. [59]

The committee also wanted to see the legislature require all local governments to regularly examine the state of the water supply and be required to provide safe water for the local inhabitants. In the 1880s and 1890s, the number of the cities with hygiene bureaus and health laboratories grew remarkably as urban officials voluntarily took up the problem of water supplies. By 1899, twenty-nine cities had health labs. [60] Many cities cooperated with the C.C.H.P. in their water investigations, and the C.C.H.P. spent much time performing examinations and going over reports in this time period. However, there were still many communes, urban and particularly rural, in which authorities took no interest in water problems. [61]

In addition to the examination of water, the committee wanted to require local officials to supply disinfection services to their citizens. Many cities were in the process of organizing such services in the 1890s. [62] The means of disinfection consisted primarily of mobile *étuves* (vaporisers) which could be brought to the locales of contagious disease. These *étuves* emitted a vapor from water heated 110-115 degrees C. and containing some antiseptic substance such as chloride, zinc or frenic acid. Some *étuves* were attached to carts which could be moved to a contaminated building for the disinfection of clothing, furniture and rugs. These articles were pushed into the top of the *étuves, as* into an oven, and then subjected to the vapor. Other *étuves* were brought into rooms where the vapor would be used to disinfect the air. These services were staffed by trained workers who would also provide residents with antiseptic solutions to scrub out floors, cupboards and walls. Many doctors and officials warned that the public would resist such draconian measures, but in fact people proved quite anxious to undergo disinfection, at least in Paris and Saint Denis. The hygiene council of the department of the Seine reported far more requests than expected for the services of their new disinfection services. In 1894 the services performed about 2,096 disinfections per arrondissement. In Paris it was noted that the poor were more cooperative than the rich. In 1906, in the XVIe arrondissement, a wealthy family complained when the local disinfection service damaged some bronze statues after several children in the family came down with the croup. However, the poor residents of the Rue Billancourt who where faced with the same croup epidemic zealously called in the service and helped with the procedures. For good measure, they performed a second fumigation themselves with sulfur. [63] Cholera was of course a prevalent reason for disinfection, but the service was also frequently called for a variety of other diseases. [64] In spite of the serious efforts made by some city officials to create such services, the C.C.H.P. noted in 1899 that most of the country, including both urban and rural areas, were without disinfection services. [65]

A very old goal of hygienists, much debated in the Academy of Medicine at this time, was the enactment of a law requiring that all residents be vaccinated against smallpox. As things stood, all school children and military men had to be vaccinated, but this meant that a substantial portion of the population escaped. Smallpox continued to cause a significant number of deaths annually in the late nineteenth century, at a rate notably higher than Britain and Germany where vaccination was required. France suffered a severe smallpox epidemic in 1870-71, and continued to suffer periodic outbreak in the 1880s and 1890s. In 1888-89 an epidemic in the Arrondissement of Pontivy in Brittany took 1034 lives out of a population of 110,000. At the commune of Douramenez in the same area there were 844 deaths among a population 10,923. [66] The debates in the Academy of Medicine focused upon the ability of the goverment to force its citizens to undergo a medical procedure. [67] In 1888 the debate was settled when a majority of the Academy voted to recommend that the legislature pass a compulsory vaccination law. However, numerous physicians remained opposed and Brouardel judged at the time that public opinion was still not ready for such a law. [68]

Finally, and perhaps most controversially, the members of the C.C.H.P. felt that two innovations were absolutely critical to the improvement of health and hygiene in France. These were the requirement of declaration of cause of death and cases of epidemic disease. These reforms were seen as crucial to maintaining an accurate picture of the status of health among the French population. The reporting of cause of death and cases of epidemic disease would alert the C.C.H.P. to the outbreak of epidemics as well as to the existence of endemic health problems. As with vaccination France was far behind the rest of Western Europe in this area of information gathering. In general, population and disease statistics were very poorly collected. In 1885 the C.C.H.P. organized a service to collect and centralize the statistics reported by cities of over 10,000 inhabitants. [69] However, this meant that only 195 urban communes reported birth, death and marriage statistics. In these communes cause of death was also reported, but because physicians were not legally required to do so, the information was quite unreliable.

The C.C.H.P. embodied most of its goals in a public law which it wrote between 1890-91 and which the government presented to the Chamber in December of 1891. The issue of pure water was embodied in another act which was presented by the government in October of 1891. The Chamber of Deputies eventually combined the two bills and discussed the law in July 1892, just after passing the Law on the Practice of Medicine (Loi Chevandier). The Public Health Law was eventually passed by the Chamber in June 1893, just before it passed the Medical Assistance Law. Therefore the years 1892 and 1893 were indeed an active period in medical legislation. Unlike the Law on Medical Assisstance and the Loi Chevandier, the Public Health Law was not immediately passed by the Senate. It languished in that house for several years and did not come up for discussion until 1897, at which time it was tabled and was not considered again until 1900. In 1901 the law passed the Senate, in modified form and was sent back to the Chamber. It was ultimately passed in 1902, in a form somewhat different from the version proposed by the C.C.H.P. in 1891, but addressing the same essential issues. [70]

The major barrier in the Senate was the Law's provisions having to do with unhealthy housing. This was the subject of much debate in that body where conservative Senators protected the interest of proprietors against a requirement that in all communes of over 20,000 population no building could be constructed without a permit. These Senators were also concerned about the provision that the local health bureaus could order the cleanup of an unhealthy habitation. The bill was ultimately passed because a compromise was worked out which Senators saw as protecting the property owner. Under this compromise, prefects and mayors, rather than the health bureaus, were to order cleanups and landlords were given a warning period and an opportunity to have a hearing. [71]

The general provisions of the Public Health Law created a public health bureaucracy, required communes to take responsible measures to stop epidemics, required the provisions of safe water, regulated unsanitary housing, mandated vaccination against smallpox, and required doctors and midwives to report cases of contagious disease. The law required all cities of 20,000 inhabitants or more, and communes of 2,000 inhabitants where there was a thermal establishment, to organize a municipal health bureau. Every department was to have a departmental health council, which would divide the department into sanitary circumscriptions. These circumscriptions would, in turn, have their own councils to oversee the communal hygiene bureaus. All communes were required to write a sanitary regulation, subject to the approval of the department health council. The departmental and sanitary circumscription councils were required to send annual reports to the C.C.H.P. on health statistics, desinfection and cleanup services.

The law obliged communal officials to take action in the case of an outbreak of contagious disease. They were required to report the outbreak to the C.C.H.P. and to use disinfecion measures, prescribed by the C.C.H.P., to stop the epidemic. Communes were also obliged to keep streets, drains, and sewers sanitary according to C.C.H.P. directives. Most importantly, all communes wee required to provide uncontaminated water to their inhabitants. Water sources were to be surrounded by a sanitary perimeter, free of disposal sites for waste, and these sites were to be covered and kept clean of polluting agents. Communes were given the right to purchase water supplies, springs and wells, through forced sale. Communes could fine people who might interfere with the programs to provide safe water. These provisions were enforced by articles which empowered the central government to force communes to comply, or to have disinfection work done, and then charge the municipal government. However, these enforcement provisions could only be put into effect if the mortality rate in a given commune exceeded the national average three years in a row or if the national government declared a state of epidemic emergency. [72]

Brouardel complained that enforcement provisions of the law, as passed, were not as strong as the C.C.H.P. had desired, and therefore was not terribly effective. The most serious change was the decision of Senators to eliminate a corps of inspectors which the C.C.H.P. had counted on to enforce the law. This corps was to have numbered 2-3,000 and been placed directly under the C.C.H.P. Bourardel also complained that the legislature refused to require salaries for the health council members at the local level. It was fear of creating more government bureaucrats which apparently caused conservatives in the Chamber and Senate to take these provisions out of the C.C.H.P.'s bill. The C.C.H.P. itself, which the law re-created under its old name of Conseil Supérieur de la Santé, was not given much authority by the law either. This situation was partially corrected by an amendment in 1906 which gave the C.C.H.P. more authority to order sanitation procedures. [73] Still, in 1906, the C.C.H.P. and the Academy of Medicine pointed out that the provisions of the law, especially the declaration of cases of epidemic disease and the organization of disinfection services, were being largely ignored outside of the major urban areas. [74]

The reaction of the Physicians' Union to the Public Health Law and related public health projects engineered by the C.C.H.P. reflected the private physicians' general anxieties about the bacteriological revolution as discussed in the first chapter. The reputation of medicine was enhanced, but the apparent drift toward increased institutionalization and bureaucratization threatened doctors. The Public Health Law was hotly discussed in Le Concours and the medical syndicat press in the period

1890-93, and again in 1897 and 1900-01. Doctors saw the provisions requiring the declaration of cases of epidemic disease, vaccination, disinfection, and the general creation of a public health bureaucracy, as hazards to the practice of medicine.

For the doctors, centralization was to be avoided at all costs. The syndicat movement argued that all public health authority should be vested in the communes and certainly not given to the department let alone the national C.C.H.P. This anti-centralization argument would also come up with regard to the Medical Assistance Law and the legislature seemed to agree with doctors on this issue in both cases. Neither program was as centralized as the committees planning them desired. The doctors' complaints about the creation of too many medical bureaucrats was also reflected by the Senate when it abolished the inspection corps. [75] In 1892, Cézilly was entirely opposed to the public health law. He claimed the law was both "too general" and "too specific." For Cézilly the limits of bureaucratic medicine were too vaguely defined and many specific provisions were harmful to private practice. [76] Union doctors were especially concerned about article eleven of the law which gave the C.C.H.P. the right to deliberate on "questions having to do with the exercise of medicine." As Gassot put it,

> "When it is a question of hygiene, of sanitation measures, of prevention, of water supplies, we have no objections ... but in the case of the exercise of medicine, does this really involve the health council?" [77]

Gassot believed that A.J. Martin, the original author of the law, had a sinister plan in mind to create a "superior council of medicine," which would have authority over the licensing and practice of doctors. As far as Gassot was concerned those whose "horizons extend only from the Arc de Triomphe to the Place de la République," had no business trying to dominate the practice of medicine. [78] In spite of Gassot's apprehensions, article eleven was in fact so vague that it had no practical effect. Some Union doctors claimed that public health could not be regulated at all, that the correct path of action was the education of public attitudes and practices: a task which should be carried out by the private physicians themselves. [79]

On the issue of smallpox vaccination, the syndicat movement had little to say about the general issue of whether or not it should be obligatory, except to note that these debates had been going on in the Academy of Medicine. However, syndicat doctors did frequently protest against the free vaccination programs which were carried out periodically at places such as the Academy of Medicine. The syndicat felt it was important, in the face of the Public Health Law, to make sure that the requirement of vaccination would not spark the spread of these free vaccination programs. Doctors in the Union movement conceded free vaccination for the destitute but demanded that all others pay private practitioners for this service. [80] The doctors' position on disinfection was similar to that on vaccination. They were concerned that they have a role in the process, and worked to make sure that in practice disinfection services were to be carried out, or at least called in, by the attending physician. [81]

The most important protest which private physicians made against the Public Health Law was the requirement that doctors, as well as *officers de santé* and midwives, report cases of contagious disease. The requirement carred fines for non-compliance. This provision was placed in the Public Health Law; however, it was first passed as part of the Loi Chevandier of 1892, a law which re-regulated to the practice of medicine and was also a subject of controversy among the syndicat movement and the C.C.H.P. A discussion of the debate over declaration of contagious disease will be presented in the following chapter which deals with the formulation of the Loi Chevandier.

In the 1890s members of the C.C.H.P. became involved in another program which ran into the opposition of syndicat doctors. Around the turn of the century tuberculosis replaced cholera and typhoid as the disease which most concerned hygienists and populationists. It was estimated that this disease caused 100,000-150,000 deaths in France each year. [82] The statistics on tuberulosis were unreliable, however, and were the subject of much discussion. Hygienists believed that tuberculosis was often misdiagnosed, sometimes unwittingly, but also deliberately by physicians anxious to protect the reputation of their clients. The mistaken diagnoses included other lung diseases such as bronchitis, broncho-pneumonia, and pleurisy. In practice, health statisticians who arrived at the commonly accepted figure of 150,000 deaths per year due to tuberculosis added in a portion of deaths attributed to chronic bronchitis. This figure of 150,000 was supported by the

Academy of Medicine, but some hygienists disputed it. It was also pointed out that doctors commonly diagnosed infantile meningitis as tuberculosis, thus inflating the statistics. In actuality true tuberculosis was rare among children ages 0-5. The anti-tuberculosis commission, organized in 1899, was quite sensitive to the common perception that France had the highest tuberculosis rate in Western Europe, and seemed to be anxious to promote lower estimates of the disease. They noted that France had developed a very bad reputation in regard to tuberculosis. Commission members, Dr. Albert Robin, Antoine Armaingaud, and Jacques Bertillon argued that tuberculosis deaths were diminishing due to better overall economic conditions and the success of preventative public health measures such as better housing, sterilized milk, and dispensary and sanatorium care. They believed that the high estimates of the Academy of Medicine were based upon the experience of hospital doctors who were seeing more tuberculosis cases. This, the commission believed, was due to the fact that more people were seeking treatment in hospitals. The commission thus rejected the estimate of 150,000 cases per year and estimated them at 100,000. [83]

Tuberculosis had long been seen as a social disease, caused by miasmas and not contagious. Thanks to the work of Koch, however, it was established that tuberculosis was contagious by means of the discharge from the lungs of the victims. In 1889, seven years after Koch's discovery, the Academy of Medicine officially declared that the disease was contagious. In 1899, Léon Bourgeois and fellow solidarist and then Premier, Waldeck-Rousseau, founded the *Commission permanente contre la tuberculose.* [84] Dr. Jacques Joseph Grancher of the C.C.H.P., Academy of Medicine, Faculty of Medicine, and Pasteur Institute, was also a member of the commission, along with Brouardel. Several important members of the C.C.H.P. were also on the anti-tuberculosis commission, including Senator Jules Siegfried, A.J. Martin, Dr. Lancereaux and Henri Monod. [85]

Brouardel and Grancher were advocates of the use of dispensaries to combat tuberculosis. They argued that for wealthy victims of tuberculosis, isolation and care was provided by the private sanatoriums which were rapidly increasing in number. However, for the poor no such institutions were available. The state could build sanatoriums and force the poor into them, as some countries had done; however, the anti-tuberculosis movement in France objected to this as not in keeping with French love of individualism and liberty. The solution backed by the C.C.H.P. and the anti-tuberculosis committee was to build dispensaries for out-patient care in urban areas where there were many working class victims living in close proximity with one another. [86] Dispensary care for tuberculosis victims had already begun at some *Bureau de bienfaisance* in the mid-1880s. [87]

The new dispensary program was first tried out in Lille where the local Pasteur Institute created an out-patient service for tuberculosis victims, called the Preventorium Emile Roux, after Pasteur's major assistant and pioneer in tuberculosis research. Lille, one of the nation's oldest and largest industrial cities, had a serious tuberculosis problem among its working class. The Pasteur Institute of Lille, under the

direction of another important tuberculosis researcher, Dr. Albert Calmette, created neighborhood dispensaries to treat victims and advise
their families. The service was modeled after a dispensary service
created in Edinburgh by Sir Robert Philip. The Lille program was
begun in 1901, at the same time that the final version of the Public
Health Law was being discussed in the legislature. The dispensaries
were sponsored by the anti-tuberculosis commission, and funded out of
the general funds of the Pasteur Institute and by a 10,000 franc grant
from the City of Lille. The main emphasis of the program was on
tuberculosis, but the dispensaries treated other lung diseases as well.
Calmette's goal was to stop contagion in the homes of the working
class victims of lung disease and improve the survival rates of those
victims. The dispensaries combined research and care, a program which
was becoming traditional with the Pasteur Institutes. The dispensary
gave out some medicines and foods to victims, but most importantly
educated the working class victims as how to sanitarily dispose of
expectorant and not contaminate their families. To this end, dispensaries also provided handkerchiefs and spitoons. [88]

The dispensary movement in Lille ran up against the deep-seated
anti-institutional orientation of private physicians and their fear of the
effects of the hygiene movement on clienteles. The Lille doctor's syndicat, already upset about the effects of the Public Health Law, saw the
dispensaries as yet another blow against their clienteles. The doctors
feared that because of the Public Health Law, they would lose clients by
being forced to report cases of tuberculosis. The doctors reasoned that

when patients realized that private care no longer assured privacy they would decide that they had nothing to lose by being treated at the dispensaries. [89] Even before the dispensaries were functioning, doctors were convinced that dispensary physicians would not confine their services to the very poor as they promised to do but would take paying clients away from neighborhood physicians. [90] The syndicat stated its position in the following terms:

> "Everyone knows that the several hundred tubercular and pre-tubercular patients that each dispensary will overfeed with public money, will be subtracted from the accounts books of the most humble neighborhood physicians." [91]

To the Lille syndicat, the expansion of the role of the Pasteur institute was ominous. The proper function of the institute, in their view, was research and the manufacture and dispensing of anti-toxins and serums. According to Lille doctors, by getting into treatment the institute was invading "...the terrain where we live." It would be better, doctors felt, if the Lille Pasteur Institute would follow the course of its sister in Bordeaux, where the institute provided consultation services to private physicians but did not serve patients directly. [92] The Lille syndicat felt that there was already more than enough institutional care available for the poor through the *bureaux de bienfaisance* and workers' insurance societies. [93]

The Syndicat complaints against the doctors of the Pasteur Institute carried a bitter tone. The syndicat doctors noted that the medical elites of Lille, represented by *l'Echo médical de Lille* and the doctors who were attached to the Pasteur Institute, were the ones who were behind the dispensaries, and that none of the private practitioners, outside of the very few who had been included in the service, supported them. The syndicat doctors also complained that the originator of the program, Dr. Albert Calmette, was also Director of the Pasteur Institute, and a professor at the Lille Faculty of Medicine, and they asked, "Didn't he already have enough to do?" [94] The public, the syndicat complained, was under the impression that those doctors connected with the Pasteur Institutes and the hygiene movement were in possession of means of curing superior to those of private physicians. Nothing could be further from the truth, according to the syndicat, and moreover these elite doctors benefited from a entirely undeserved prestige. The syndicat implied that the hygienist movement misled the public. They pointed out that there had been a great deal of publicity given to the supposed discovery of an anti-tuberculosis vaccine (by Koch). When this vaccine proved useless, hygienists had been very reticent about discussing it in public. However the hygienists continued to print up fancy brochures advising the public on the prevention of tuberculosis and, the syndicat claimed, hygienists manipulated statistics to prove the efficacy of the preventative measures they advocated. [95]

The dispensaries apparently tried to be careful to treat only those patients who were registered as eligible for care at the free medical services of the local *bureau de bienfaisance*. This was not enough for the syndicat, however. The syndicat put great pressure upon Dr. Calmette to disassociate the dispensaries from the Pasteur Institute and therefore to make sure the dispensaries did not fall under the aura of the name

Pasteur. They also demanded that neighborhood doctors be employed at the dispensaries. The Lille syndicat marshalled its forces by obtaining the support of the four other large medical syndicats in the area, those at Roubaix, Douai, Armentieres and Tourcoing which were anxious not to see the dispensary idea spread to their cities. Calmette bowed to the pressure and agreed to separate the dispensaries from the Pasteur Institute, both administratively and physically. Even though Calmette acquiesced to their demand, the syndicat continued to grumble that he was just complying in "appearance." [96]

The Lille syndicat had the support of the Seine physicians' syndicat and the Union of Syndicats. The Union maintained that the Lille dispensaries were "without notable effect," and also "conflicted with our major goal of leaving patients to their doctors as much as possible." [97] The problem in Lille, according to the Union, was that the dispensaries had not been planned in conjunction with local doctors but had been sprung upon them unawares. In Bordeaux, by contrast, the syndicat doctors had been consulted from the very beginning with the result that the anti-tuberculosis services of the Pasteur Institute were being provided in a way which Lille doctors believed was satisfactory to all. The Union and the Seine syndicat agreed with their brothers in Lille that the Pasteur institutes should stick to research, serum and consultation services for doctors and stay out of practice. [98]

The Pasteur institutes' role in providing serums to private physicians was not without conflict either. By the turn of the century the institutes were providing serums against diphtheria, one of the first successful serums to be developed. In 1901, however, Waldeck-Rousseau sent a notice to health boards and institutes noting the fact that physicians often used the anti-diphtheria serum too late to be effective; as a result diphtheria deaths were on the rise again. This notice was given publicity in *Le Matin* and *l'Eclair*. The Union and the syndicats of the Seine and of Lille were angered by this publicity. The Seine syndicat commented that this would encourage parents to sue their doctors in court for misuse of anti-diphtheria serum, even when their child had actually died from the croup. In Lille, doctors saw this as another effort of the Pasteur Institute to tarnish the reputation of private doctors. [99]

Other programs of the anti-tuberculosis commission also ran into difficulties from local doctors. Around 1903 Dr. Grancher began to place Parisian children from tuberculosis-contaminated environments in the homes of rural residents. The children were healthy and Grancher's goal was to prevent them from catching the disease. Also, by following their progress, he hoped to make some observations about the role of heredity versus contagion in the disease. The families with whom the children were placed were paid twenty-five to thirty francs per month. However, in Nogent-sur-Seine, where five children were placed, the local sanitary commission protested their presence. Under the advice of the local commission, the villagers ostracized the children, not allowing them in school or church. The local sanitary commission sent a petition to the anti-tuberculosis commission claiming that the commission was purposfully trying to convert the healthy village into a "tuberculosis den," for the purposes of experimentation. Grancher blamed the local doctors for inciting the residents, who otherwise, he believed, would have been glad of the economic benefits of the generous government money comming into the area. The prefect backed up the villagers and requested that the children be withdrawn. [100]

Grancher admitted that part of the reasons for the program were "the interests of science," but claimed that the local doctors had no scientific basis for their fears. Grancher did agree that the children would no longer attend school. As this affair became known, other rural doctors began to protest against Grancher's program. [101] Clearly, Grancher was doing exactly what Bourgeois had argued against in his 1889 address to the C.C.H.P., using the public as a terrain of experimentation. In stopping the program, local doctors were trying to protect their local communities albeit in a misguided fashion. However, in working against the dispensary program in Lille, it is difficult to see how doctors were protecting anyone but themselves.

The bacteriological revolution brought more conflict to an already divided medical establishment. Hygienists, drawn mostly from the medical elites, were at last able to offer really effective solutions to the nation's worst disease problems, typhoid and cholera. Moreover, the hygienists could clearly demonstrate that the disinfection of water supplies and sanitary disposal of sewage could have a dramatic impact on the major epidemic diseases. No private medical practitioners, licensed or otherwise, could demonstrate such efficacy. Thus there was no doubt that really effective medical techniques lay in the realm of prevention, rather than treatment. Prevention, in the form of public health regulations, however, was not in keeping with the professional image of practitioners in the Union movement. Their self-concepts and livelihoods were dependent upon treatment, the direct intervention of the individual practitioner after disease had already struck. Thus when faced with the implications of the bacteriological revolution, the private practitioners never questioned the justification for the continuation of private practice as the dominant form of medical care. Rather, they worked assiduously through the Union movement to preserve and promote the traditional, private, and non-preventative, nature of medical care. The bacteriological revolution did not provide a concept around which to unify a profession; rather it provided a challenge to the pre-existing professional concepts. For the mass of practitioners professionalization occurred as the result of a movement which supported traditional medical roles against public health. Practitioners were quite willing to call themselves hygienists, basking in the reflected glory of Pasteur and the other great scientists of the age. But the were not willing to countenance any public health reform which involved the intervention of the state into the private practice of medicine.

Organized into their Union movement, the private pactitioners were more than a match for the C.C.H.P. and other public health organizations. The Union movement successfully reduced the scope of the dispensary movement, making sure the dispensaries would generally only support the private treatment of tuberculosis and other contagious diseases, rather than treat patients directly. Further, the movement put limits on the treatment of patients at hospitals. Doctors refused to cooperate in the reporting of cases of contagious disease and in their reporting of health statistics. They successfully resisted the creation of a strong, centralized public health bureaucracy.

As Léon Bourgeois so carefully explained, state intervention in the form of public health was part of the solidarist program to defend the health of the nation against the menace of contagion and resulting depopulation. There was no groundswell of popular resistance against this form of state intervention; on the contrary, dispensaries, free vaccination services and disinfection services were welcomed and widely utilized by the public. The opposition to intervention in the form of public health came from special interests groups: landlords and private practitioners in the Union movement. In medical legislation in this period, the support or opposition of doctors in the Union movement was crucial. The Medical Practice Law (*Loi Chevandier*), Medical Assistance Law and Public Health Law were all supported by solidarists. The Public Health Law was largely opposed by the doctors' Union movement and thus was delayed and ultimately stripped of effectiveness during its course through the legislature. However, the Medical Practice and Medical Assistance Laws, strongly supported by the Union movement, moved quickly the legislature and were enacted a full decade before the eviscerated public health act.

NOTES TO CHAPTER II

1. George Rosen, *A History of Public Health,* pp 282-330. Rosen points out that in the eighteenth century, most medical men believed in a combination of contagion and miasma.

2. Erwin Ackerknecht. "Anti-contagionism 1821-1887," *Bulletin of the History of Medicine* V. 22 (1948), p 562.

3. W. Barry Wood, *From Miasmas to Molecules.*

4. W. Barry Wood, *Ibid*

5. Pierre Bretonneau produced a microbial theory of diphtheria in 1821; Agnostino Bassi did the same for silkworm disease in the 1830s; John Snow for cholera in the 1850s; William Budd for typhoid in 1873; Semmelweiss for peuperal fever in 1849 and, working independently, Holmes for the same disease in 1855: W. Barry Wood, *Ibid*

6. Ann Elizabeth Fowler La Berge, "Public Health in France and the French Public Health Movement, 1815-1848," unpublished dissertation, University of Tennessee, March 1874, p 117.

7. La Berge, *Ibid,* pp 120-127; Ackerknecht, *Ibid.*

8. La Berge, *Ibid;* also by the same author, "The French Public Health Movement, 1815-1848," *Proceedings of the Western Society for French*

History 1977.

9. Rosen Ibid.; Ackerknecht Ibid.

10. Bernard-Pierre Lecuyer, "Médecins et observateurs sociaux: Les Annales d'Hygiène publique et de médecine légale, (1820-1850)", *Pour une histoire de la statistique* , V. 8.

11. AN f8 170; .

12. Brouardel, *La Profession médicale*, 1903 pp 61-65.

13. AN F8 170.

14. R.C.C.H.P., V. 2 (Part II) (1882) pp 66-73. R.C.C.H.P., V 19, (1889), pp 517-520.

15. R.C.C.H.P., V. 12 (Part II), (1882) p 70.

16. P. Brouardel, "Taux de mortalité 1893-1898," R.C.C.H.P., 1900, pp 86-89; Dr. A. Alison, *Etiologie de la Fièvre typhoide dans les campagnes*, 1880.

17. R.C.C.H.P., V. 19 (1889), pp 325; V. 18 (1888), pp 207.

18. AN F8 170; R.C.C.H.P., V. 19, pp 322-339.

19. Mc Innes, Mary Elizabeth *Essentials of Communicable Diseases* , 1975.

20. Rosen, *Ibid*

21. Drs. Bouchardat, Colin, Voisin, "Rapport sur la nécessité d'isoler les enfants atteints de la rougeole et autres maladies contagieuses," AD XIX S 25.

22. He was made an "auditeur" in 1884.

23. A.J. Martin, "Organisation de la médecine publique en France," *Annales d'hygiène publique, industrielle et sociale,* Vol. 7 (1882), pp 213-271; Vol 9 (1883) pp 137-152; "Essai d'organisation de la médecine publique en France, " *Revue d'hygiène et de police sanitaire ,* V. II (1880).

24. R.C.C.H.P., V. 19, (1889), pp i-viii.

25. *Ibid*

26. Macfarlane Burnet, *The Natural History of Infectious Disease* 1953; Napias and Martin, *l'Hygiène en France* R.C.C.H.P. Tables-Répertoires 1872-1890.

27. Dr. Ollivier, "Rapport sur la Fièvre typhoide à Paris et sa prophylaxie," *Conseil d'hygiène publique et de salubrité du département de la Seine;* AD XIX S 24; R.C.C.H.P. V. 20 (1890), pp 389-390.

28. Dr. L.H. Thoinot, "Fièvre typhoide en France: Etiologie et Prophalaxie - Etude de quelques foyers de fièvre typhoide en France," R.C.C.H.P., V. 20 (1890) pp 380-407.

29. P. Brouardel et Dr. Chantemesse, "l'Epidémie de Fièvre typhoide qui a regne à Clermont-Ferrand - 1886."

30. Dr. L.H. Thoinot, *Ibid.*

31. Dr. A. Alison, *Etiologie de la Fièvre typhoide dans les campagnes,* 1880.

32. A. Durand-Claye, "l'Epidémie de Fièvre typhoide à Paris en 1882," *Journal de la Société de la Statistique de Paris.*

33. Dr. A. Alison, *Ibid.*

34. In the midst of the continuing controversy over whether contagious diseases were caused by organic or inorganic substances the hygienists were given to using the more ambiguous term "principe morbifique." see P. Brouardel *Fièvre typhoide des Modes de Propagation,* 1887; Dr. Ollivier, *Ibid.*

35. P. Brouardel, *Fièvre typhoide des Modes de Propagation,* 1887; Brouardel et Thoinot, *Deux épidémies de Fièvre typhoide, Annales d'hygiène,* 1891; R.C.C.H.P., V. 21 (1891); actually there was validity to some of Brouardel's claims, it is possible for the typhoid bacillus, salmonella typhosa, to transmitted by unwashed hands. The bacillus can also be transmitted by the skins of uncooked fruits and vegetables: Mc Innes, *Ibid.*

36. R.C.C.H.P., V. 21 (1891).

37. P. Brouardel, *Fièvre typhoide des Modes de Propagation.* 1887.

38. Tardieu et.al, "Instructions générales concernant les mesures préventives à prendre contre le cholera,: R.C.C.H.P. 1874, V. III, pp 316-329.

39. R.C.C.H.P., V. 21 (1892).

40. R.C.C.H.P., V. 15 (1885), p 561. The death statistics probably greatly underestimate the actual deaths because most communes simply did not keep track of the number of deaths let alone their causes.

41. The *Maison départementale* at Nanterre was a prison and *Dépôt de Mendacité* (home for indigents) for the department of the Seine.

42. Dr. Dujardin-Beaumetz, "l'Epidémie cholerique en 1892 dans le Département de la Seine," (based upon the investigations of Thoinot and Dubief) *Conseil d'Hygiène et de Salubrité de Département de la Seine* , 1893, AN AD XIX s26; Durjardin-Beaumetz and Thoinot were both also members of the C.C.H.P., Brouardel also produced a summary of the critical Nanterre investigation in the R.C.C.H.P.: V. 22, Annex, 1892.

43. Dr. Dujardin-Beaumetz, *Ibid.*

44. Brouardel, "Le Cholera en 1892," *R.C.C.H.P.*, V. 22 Annex, 1892.

45. R.C.C.H.P., V. 18, (1888), pp 230-235; V. 22, Annex, (1892), pp xxx-3.

46. Gerard Jacquemet, "Médecine et Maladies populaires dans le Paris de la fin du XIX siècle," *Récherches* , No 29, Dec. (1977) pp 349-364; A. Chervin, "Louis Adolphe Bertillon," *Journal de la Société de la Statistque de Paris,* V. 24 (1883). The medical press also made much of depopulation fears. *Le Concours,* V. 10, N. 20, (Mars 19, 1988); *Le Courrier médical,* N. 19 (May 9, 1891),; N. 18, (May 2, 1891); *Gazette médicale de Paris,* S. 7, V. 8, N. 11, (Mar 14, 1891); *La France médicale,* V. 38, N. 45 (Nov. 6, 1891); *Gazette Hebd. des Sciences médicales de Bordeaux,* Mar. 15, 1891); see also M. Boudet, "Le Mouvement de la population en france", *Revue Scientifique* , V. 4, (June 29, 1867).

47. P. Brouardel et Dr. Chantemesse, *l'Epidémie de Fièvre typhoide que a regne à Clermont-Ferrand - 1886.*

48. "Le Cholera en 1892, preface par P. Brouardel," R.C.C.H.P., V 22, Annex (1892), p xiv.

49. M. Schutzenberger, "Rapports sur les eaux distribuées à Meudon," Conseil d'hygiène et de salubrité de la Département de la Seine: AN Ad XIX s 24.

50. Larson, *Ibid.* p 103; "Simple question à messieurs les members du Conseil d'Hygiène," *Lyon médical*, N. 4, (Jan. 27, 1878), pp 135-137.

51. Léonard, "Les Débuts du 'Concours médical'," *Histoire des Science médicales,* 1980, pp 454-55.

52. Dr. Garnier, "Gazette du Village," (Feb. 2, 1890) p 56.

53. "Le remède de Koch," *Le Concours,* V. 13, N. 4, (Jan. 24, 1891), pp 37-39; Léonard, *Ibid*

54. Paul Hastings, *Medicine, An International History,* 1974.

55. See Hoarce Bianchon, (pseud. for Maurice de Fleury), *Nos Grandes Médecins d'Audjourd'hui,* 1891.

56. Maurice de Fleury, (exerpt from article published in *Figaro,* entitled "guerre aux microbes,") *Le Concours,* V. 12, N. 40, (Oct. 4, 1890), p 476.

57. Cézilly, *Ibid.*

58. Brouardel, *La Profession médicale,*

59. A.J. Martin, "Essai d'organisation de la Médecine publique en France," *Revue d'hygiène et de police sanitaire,* Vol. II (1880) p 569; "Organisation de la médecine publique en France. Création d'une

direction de la Santé publique," *Annales d'hygiène, industrielle et sociale,* Vol 9. S. 3 (1883), p 136; "Organisation de la médecine publique en france," *Ibid.,* Vol 7. s. 3 (1882), p 213.

60. R.C.C.H.P., V. 30, (1900).

61. Georges Chalot, *Les Bureaux d'hygiène en France,* 1906; Leon Baudin, *Etat sanitaire à Besançon,* 1893; Louis Reverchon, *Création d'une Bureau d'hygiène à Lyon,* 1882; F. Coreil, *Rapport sur les travaux exécutés au Laboratoire Municipale pendant 1896 et 1897* (Toulon), 1898; M. Jeannot, *Assainissement de la Ville de Besançon et Mise à l'abri des Inodations,* 1907; *Lyon médical,* N. 5 (Feb. 1891).

62. Jules de Crisenoy, "Appareills de désinfection," *Questions d'Assistance publique traitées dans les Conseils généraux en 1893,* (hereinafter *Questions),* pp 229-259; "Services de désinfection" *Questions* 1894, pp 206-220.

63. D. Guede, "Rapport sur les travaux de la Commission d'hygiène de XVI Arrondissement pendant l'année 1900" *Réceuil des Travaux de Commission permanente contre la Tuberculose en France* (hereinafter, R.C.P.C.T.), (May 1906), pp 183-184.

64. Dr. LeRoy Barnes, "Rapport sur les maladies épidémiques et les maladies virulentes observées dans l'Arrondissement de Saint Denis," *Conseil d'hygiène et de Salubrité de la département de la Seine* AD XIX S 25.

65. R.C.C.H.P., V. 30 (1900), pp 237-239.

66. Brouardel, *La Profession médicale*

67. *Gazette Hebd. des Sciences médicales de Bordeaux* , N. 8 (Feb. 22, 1891); For a history of the politics of smallpox vaccination in France see: Jean-Noel Biraben, "La Diffusion de la Vaccination en France au XIXe siècle," *Annales de Bretagne* , V. 86, N. 2 (June 1979), pp 265-276.

68. Brouardel, *Ibid.*

69. R.C.C.H.P., V. 18, (1888), p 411.

70. *Journal Officiel* (hereinafter, J.O.), 1902, pp 98-111; R.C.C.H.P., V. 21 (1891), pp 353-453, 861-941.

71. Brouardel, *Ibid.*

72. R.C.C.H.P., *Ibid,* Brouardel, *La Profession Médicale;* J.O., *Ibid*

73. Brouardel, *Ibid;* Fernand Widal, "Rapport général à M. le Président du Conseil, Ministre de l'Intérieur, sur les épidémies en 1906," *Bull de l'Academie de Médecine* , N. 24 (June 15, 1908).

74. Widal, *Ibid*

75. *Le Concours,* V. 14, N. 2, p 13.

76. *Ibid.*

77. Gassot, "La protection de la santé publique," *Le Concours,* V. 14, N. 31 (July 30, 1892), pp 368-370.

78. *Ibid*

79. J. Noir, "l'Application de la loi sur la protection de la santé publique," *Bulletin de l'Union des Syndicats* , N. 1, (Jan. 1903), pp 18-20.

80. M. Dromain, "Contre l'état vaccinateur" *Bul. des Soc. méd. d'Arron.),* V. 3, N. VII, (April 5, 1900), p 268; Dr. Jamier, " *Bul. des syn. méd. du Nord et de Pas-de-Calais* N. 10, (Oct. 1902) pp 129-130.

81. *Le Concours,* V. 13, N. 51, (Dec. 19, 1891); *Revue des Etablissements de Bienfaisance,* V. 1895, p 32.

82. R.C.P.C.T. (Dec., 1905) p 40.

83. Dr. Armaingaud, "Décroissance de la tuberculose pulmonaire a Paris pendant les seizes années, 1888-1903, dans la population totale," R.C.P.C.T. V. 2, 1905-06; R.C.P.C.T., June 1900.

84. Yvonne Knibiehler, "La Lutte anti-tuberculeuse," *Annales de Bretagne,* V. 86, N. 2, pp 321-322.

85. R.C.P.C.T., V. 1, (1903-05).

86. Brouardel, Grancher, "Sanatoriums, la lutte contre la tuberculose," *Revue d'hygiène et de Police Sanitaire,* V. 1899, p 739; "Les sanatoriums et leurs variétés nécessaires," *Annales d'hygiène et de médecine légale* (July 1899), p 5; "A propose de la lutte contre la tuberculose, Le discours de M. le Senateur Peyrot, *Bul. de l'Union,* N. 7, (April 5, 1903).

87. Dr. Ollivier, "Médecine gratuite," *Conseil d'hygiène et de Salubrité publique de la Seine,* 1887, AD XIX s 25.

88. Dr. Paul Petite, "Visite à l'Institute Pasteur de Lille", *Bulletin officiel des Soc. méd. d'arrondissement et de Con. Gén. des Soc. du Départ. de la Seine,* V. 4, N. 111, (Feb. 5, 1901), pp 91-92; "La Nouvelle loi sur la protection de la santé publique," *Bul. de Syn. Med.*

du Nord et de Pas-de-Calais, N. 1, (Jan. 1901); *Histoire générale de la médecine,* pp 214-218; 499-501.

89. *Ibid.*

90. *Ibid.* Dr. Paul Petit, *Ibid.*

91. Drs. Boutry, Lambin, and Quint, "Les Dispensaires anti-tuberculeux," *Bul. du Syn. méd. du Nord et de Pas-de-Calais,* V. 4 (April 1901). pp 49-51.

92. "Le Conflit médical à Lille," *Bul. des syn. méd. de France,* (June 1901), p 1075.

93. Drs. Boutry, Lambin and Quint, *Ibid.*

94. *Bul. des Syn. méd. du Nord et de Pas-de-Calais,* N. 6 (June, 1901), p 85.

95. *Ibid.;* Dr. Coppens, *Bul. des syn. méd. du Nord et de Pas-de-Calais,* N. 5, (May 1901), pp 63; N. 6, (June, 1901); N. 8, (August, 1901) p 120.

96. Drs. A. Coppens, Declercq, Defaux, Douche, Lambin, Lefebvre, "Les Dispensaires et l'Institut Pasteur de Lille," *Bul. des Syn. méd du Nord et de Pas-de-Calais,* N. 6 (June 1, 1901), pp 80-83; N. 7 (July, 1901).

97. *Bul. des Syn. méd. de France,* (June, 1901) p 1075.

98. *Ibid.;* Dr. Jamier, Président du Syndicat des médecins de la Seine, "Lettre", *Bul. des Syn. méd. du Nord et de Pas-de-Calais, N. 10,* (Oct. 1901), pp 129-130.

99. *Bul. des Syn. méd. du Nord et de Pas-de-Calais,* N. 7, (July, 1901).

100. *R.C.P.C.T.,* (May 1906), pp 181-199.

101. *Ibid.*

CHAPTER III

THE LOI CHEVANDIER

Union doctors recognized that the late 1880s and early 1890s offered new opportunities as well as new dangers to the profession. Although the public health movement was threatening their terrain of practice, the enhanced prestige of medicine brought by that same movement could benefit private physicians. In addition, the concerns of the solidarist-populationist program meant that the political climate was right for medical legislation. These two factors created an atmosphere more receptive to the demands of the profession than ever before in the history of French medicine. Doctors in the Union movement were aware of these developments and were quite adept at manipulating populationist and solidarist concerns to their own advantage. Further, they specifically noted and discussed how the bacteriological revolution might be used to promote their own professional goals. Populationist concerns were used by the Union in an effective lobbying campaign aimed at the legislature and the public health bureaucracy. This campaign resulted in the passage of a long-desired new law on the practice of medicine, the Loi Chevandier. At the same time that the syndicat was working on this project, it was also promoting another piece of legislation, the Medical Assistance Law of 1893, a subject which will be taken up in the next chapter. The Loi Chevandier and the Medical Assistance Law, both traveled a much smoother path in the Legislature than the Public Health Law which was being considered at the same time. Thus the two laws sponsored by the Union movement were passed by the legislature in 1892 and 1893 while the public health legislation was delayed for another decade.

The Law Chevandier was passed by the Chamber in 1891 and by the Senate in 1892 and was supported by the Left Republican-Radical governments of Charles Floquet and Pierre Tirard, and ultimately by the Moderate governments of Charles Louis Freycinet, and Emile Loubet. In general, the law had broad support from all sectors of republican politics; however, a few voices of protest were raised against certain provisions. These voices came from both the conservative right and from the republican left. In addition, there were major differences in the text of the law as drafted by the syndicat and as drafted by the C.C.H.P. These conflicts were eventually worked out between the two groups, in a way which favored private physicians. The general provisions of the law were as follows: the gradual destruction of the *officiate de santé;* further restrictions on the practice of midwives; the legalization of physicians' syndicats; the strengthening of the definition of illegal practice and of the penalties against it; provisions which helped physicians in the collection of fees; and the requirement of physicians to declare cases of contagious disease to public authorities. These measures, with the exception of the reporting of cases of epidemic disease, were great victories for the newly formed physicians' Union. The law largely determined the shape of the modern medical care system.

Union doctors were quite sensitive to the changes taking place in the public image of medicine as a result of the bacteriological revolution. The medical press took note of the fact that for the first time scientific developments in medicine were being reported in the regular press and were receiving tremendous public attention and acclaim. [1] The Union of syndicats and *Le Concours* consciously set out to take advantage of the improved reputation of scientific medicine to solve what they perceived as the crisis facing the profession. Dr. Aymard of the Union put the issue quite plainly:

"the new role that [the doctor] is called upon to play in modern society offers him rewards which, if he knows how to take advantage of them as he should, will permit him to escape victoriously from the current medical crisis and to reconquer the role ... that the medical family is in danger of losing altogether." [2]

The Union movement also took note of the fact that the large numbers of doctors in the legislature offered a fruitful source for the advancement of professional goals. There were fifty physician-deputies and senators in 1888, and eighty after the legislative elections of 1889. In 1893, fourteen physician-legislators were members of *Le Concours*. [3] However, Union leaders recognized that the help of these doctor-politicians was not always readily forthcoming. Dr. Aymard warned that the Union movement should not put too much faith in the *médecins-députés* who, with a few outstanding exceptions, usually forgot they were doctors as soon as they entered the legislature. More important to the Union was the influence they themselves could bring to bear on the legislature and bureaucracy. Doctors took note of the fact that the legislature had been behaving as if new hygiene services would be performed by physicians free of charge. The syndicat set out to correct this view and to assure that doctors would receive proper compensation for the new role they were being asked to play in society. [4] In the eyes of the Union movement, this compensation should consist of state recognition and support for professional goals in the form of favorable legislation.

At its general assembly in October of 1889, the members of *Le Concours* set out their lobbying program and legislative goals in frank terms. Examining the question of "how to influence the legislature," Dr. Fourmestreaux noted that they would have to use their influence on all deputies, not just physician-deputies. [5] At that meeting, Union pointed to Deputies Chevandier and David as their main sources of support in the Chamber. Bragging that the Union leaders "already had the ear of the government," Dr. Jeanne, the secretary of the Union, said that the next step was to get specific commitments from as many deputies as possible to support a new law on the exercise of medicine and a law on medical public assistance. Further, the Union movement should put pressure on "false-doctors," those in positions of power who did not support their professional goals. [6] Jeanne pointed out that 1889 was a landmark year in the history of medical care in France because in January ministerial changes went into effect which revitalized the public health bureaucracy. By placing the Public Assistance Council (C.S.A.P.- *Conseil supérieur de l'Assistance publique)* and the C.C.H.P. under the same ministry and director, state health care programs were for the first time unified under one administration. These changes were an indication of government recognition of the importance of health issues. Jeanne explained that public assistance and public health were thus becoming important areas for syndicat action to achieve professional goals. He argued,

"Is it not just that the men who constitute their personnel should become recognized but also that they should be put into possession of the means to live in accordance with the other professions?" [7]

Jeanne told the members of *Le Concours* that a law on the exercise of medicine, giving doctors a stronger monopoly and more financial security, was required of the French legislature if it truly desired to see France become the equal of other modern nations in public health. This was the line of argument which *Le Concours* used in support of the Loi Chevandier; however, it was never made clear how increasing the doctors' monopoly over medical practice would benefit public health. Among themselves, on the other hand, doctors in the Union movement noted that the Loi Chevandier would help to overcome their problems of oversupply of physicians, competition with illegal practitioners, and difficulties in collecting fees.

The Union leaders were quite aware that their aggressive quest for beneficial legislative action risked worsening the bad image of doctors. Dr. Gibert cautioned against exposing their professional goals to the public and recommended avoiding the attention of the popular press as much as possible. The Union was careful to confine its activities to the profession, legislature and bureaucaracy. [8] In addition, the Union, according to Fourmestreaux's explicit policy, cultivated a "humanitarian" image by sending representatives to international health conferences. At those conferences the representatives were instructed to be careful not to raise issues pertaining to professional interests. [9]

Just a few weeks after the October 20, 1889 Assembly of *Le Concours,* Deputy Chevandier proposed a revision of the 1803 law on medical practice to the Chamber. [10] This version of the law was backed by *Le Concours* and the Union, and was based upon a draft of a new law which had been produced by the Medical Congress of 1845. At that time a new law on the practice of medicine had been proposed by the Minister of Education, Salvandy. This law was passed by the Chambre des Pairs in 1847 but was buried in the furor of 1848. [11]

The efforts of Chevandier and others to see a new law on the practice of medicine passed went back to the early Third Republic. In 1871, Chevandier submitted his first proposed version for a new law. The A.G.M.F. then took up the issue, but their many discussions came to nothing. Finally in the 1880s the issue was taken up by *Le Concours* in association with Chevandier. In 1883 the opportunist government of Jules Ferry made a commitment to medical reform and charged Chevandier to head a committee to write a law. In 1885, Chevandier reported on the committee's work, and the de Freycinet government of 1886 asked the C.C.H.P. to study the issue. The C.C.H.P. wrote its own version which was presented in 1886. However, the Chamber ignored the C.C.H.P. version and accepted the Chevandier version intact. In 1889, after the legislative elctions, Chevandier and the C.C.H.P., both reintroduced their versions of the law. Again the Chevandier version was accepted for consideration, with one important change, the addition of an article on the declaration of contagious disease. [12] The C.C.H.P. project differed in several respects from that proposed by Chevandier. Between 1889 and 1891, when the project was ultimately considered by the Chamber, the Chevandier committee and the C.C.H.P. attempted to work out a compromise version of the law. During this period, *Le Concours* put considerable pressure on the public health bureaucracy to accept their version of the law.

The abolition of the *officiers de santé* was the subject of a major quarrel between the advocates of the Chevandier and C.C.H.P. versions of the law. As was noted in Chapter I, the *officiers* were intended to consitute a corps of practitioners for rural France. [13] In order to keep them confined to local areas, the territory of their practice was limited to the department in which they were awarded their degree. The nature of their practice was identical to that of the *docteur,* except that they were not allowed to perform major surgery without the supervision of a *docteur.* [14] In actuality, in most of France there was little distinction in the popular mind between *docteurs* and *officiers* and many of the latter were, like Charles Bovary of Flaubert's novel, addressed by their patients as "doctor médecin." [15] The officiate became a very popular profession for sons of the lower middle class during the early part of the century. By 1847 there were, according to the C.C.H.P., 7,456 of them practicing in the nation, thus making up about forty per cent of all licensed general medical practitioners. (See Table I-1). [16] After 1847 the number of *officiers* declined rapidly; there were only 2,512 of them, or fourteen per cent of total licensed general medical practitioners, in 1881. No doubt the *officiers* were hurt more than the *docteurs* by the effects of oversupply. However, the decline of the *officiers* was caused at least in part by efforts on the part of the *docteurs* to reduce their numbers. Educational reforms in the training of the *officiers de santé* in 1856 and 1883, put into effect at the request of the professors at the Faculties of medicine, made the degree of *officers de santé* more difficult to obtain. Also the educational changes (discussed in Chapter I) made it easier to obtain a place at a medical faculty and no doubt made the officiate less attractive.

If the number of *officiers* was declining anyway, why were doctors so concerned with abolishing them? Doctors of the Union movement were very concerned about the unity of the profession. They wanted to see all practitioners become as equal as possible. Therefore they worked toward the elimination of the lower orders of general practitioners, the *officiers,* as well as to reduce those factors which created the medical elites. In the short run they very much needed the support of the officiers to promote their professional goals. *Officiers* moreover, were syndicat and Union members. Therefore the Union draft of the Medical Practice Law, provided that those *officiers* in practice and those students for the degree of officiate be allowed to practice until the end of their lives. It also recommended that the *officiers* be allowed to receive a *doctorate* with a relatively simple examination. The doctors' anxieties about the *officiers* seems also to have been aroused by the fear that the officiate was about to expand again. In fact it is apparent that based upon the number of diplomas issued, the officiate was beginning to recover between 1882 and 1884. This increase in diplomas was obscured by the statistics on the total number of *officiers,* taken at five year intervals. The effects of this increase in diplomas would not have made an impact on the total number of *officiers* practicing until after 1892. In the meantime the Loi Chevandier was passed and many students for the officiate took advantage of the provisions made in that law for them to become *docteurs.*

Initially the C.C.H.P strongly disapproved of the plans of Chevandier and the syndicat movement to abolish the *officiers de santé.* The C.C.H.P. had supported the officiate for some time out of concern over the severe shortage of practitioners in some parts of the nation. In 1890, the sub-committee of the C.C.H.P. which supported the continutation of the officiate, and opposed that section of the Chevandier bill which would abolish them, contained most of the important hygienists in the nation. [17] In 1873, the C.C.H.P. had recommended regulations to make it easier for *officiers* to transfer between departments, with the explicit hope that this would help spread practitioners to undersupplied areas. [18] In 1886, in its report on the Chevandier bill, the C.C.H.P. reiterated this position. The health committee explicitly argued to the government that the *officiers* were needed to assure that licensed practitioners would be available to the entire population. The committee noted that when the number of *officiers* was at its height in 1847, the ratio of practitioners to population was also probably at its highest point of the century (about one per 1898 inhabitants). [19] Between 1847 and 1881, the most recent census year at the time of the C.C.H.P. report, the ratio of practitioners to inhabitants had steadily declined (to one per 2,536 inhabitants). [20] The C.C.H.P. also pointed out that as of 1881, five-sixths of all communes in the nation were without resident practitioners. Further, the number of communes without resident practitioners had increased by about one hundred since 1876. [21]

The C.C.H.P. noted that while it was true that many *officiers,* like *docteurs,* were concentrated in urban communes, the statistics on the distribution of medical practitioners showed that *officiers* were, to a significant degree, fulfilling the role envisioned for them in 1803 as rural practitioners. Of course, the fact that the *officiers* were prevented from establishing practices outside the departments in which they were trained kept them out of many poor under-medicalized departments which did not have medical schools. This was particularly true after the educational change of 1853 took the examination of the *officiers* away from departmental juries and gave it to examination boards at the medical schools themselves. This effectively prevented *officiers* from practicing in departments without medical schools.

The C.C.H.P. believed that if the *officiers* were abolished, *docteurs* would not step in to replace them. The health committee could point to some revealing statistics to support this contention. In 1866 thirteen departments had an excess of *officiers* over docteurs. Of these thirteen, by 1881 all had shown a great decline in the number of *officiers* with no corresponding increase in the number of *docteurs*. [22] The supporters of the officiate argued that abolishing them would open up the country-side to hordes of charlatans and stop the progress of vaccination against smallpox. These were precisely the dangers that the Union movement purported to be working against. [23] C.C.H.P. members pointed out that the two grades of practitioners were drawn from different social groups: the *docteurs* from the upper bourgeoisie; the *officiers* from the petty bourgeoisie, "artisans, de petits commercants, de petits proprietaires agricoles, de contre maitres." [24] The families of the *officiers* were those who could not afford the more expensive secondary education and more lengthy medical training required of the *docteurs,* but who still aspired to see their sons placed in a profession. The offspring of such families, the committee believed, were far more willing than the sons of the bourgeoisie to live out their lives in isolated rural communes. More-over, the committee felt it was socially just to reserve this channel of social mobility for the sons of artisans, small businessmen and peasant land owners. The committee concluded that to abolish the *officiers* was to close a whole class of society off from medical careers.

Besides recommending the continuation of the officiate, the C.C.H.P. wanted to use the new law to improve the status of the *officiers* and increase their medical prerogatives. The committee wanted to abolish the two limitations on the practice of *officiers* made by the law of 1803 so the *officiers* would be free to set up practice in any department and could perform surgery without supervision. This would make them the virtual equals of the *docteurs*. [25]

Between 1886 and 1890, the Union movement succeeded in changing the opinions of the C.C.H.P. on the *officiers de santé*. The key figure in this change of view was Paul Brouardel, president of the C.C.H.P. (see Chapter I). In 1873, before joining the C.C.H.P., Brouardel supported the A.G.M.F. in advocating the abolition of the officiate. [26] In 1886-88, after joining the C.C.H.P., he became an ardent supporter of the officiate. Brouardel argued that contrary to the view of the Union doctors, having two grades of medical practitioners was not undemocratic. At this time, Brouardel shared the opinion expressed by the C.C.H.P., that the officiate served a useful purpose that could not readily be met by *docteurs*. Moreover, he argued that *docteurs* would lose prestige by practicing in the backward rural villages served by the *officiers*. [27]

By 1890 Brouardel had altered his view dramatically and again began to call for the abolition of the officiate. He repeated the same arguments used by the Union: there were too many practitioners and that having two grades of practitioners was undemocratic. Some *officiers de santé* and their supporters felt Brouardel had betrayed them. They pointed out that the 1886 C.C.H.P. report, co-authored by Brouardel, had provided convincing statistics on the usefulness of the officiate. How then, they asked, could Brouardel, "who had defended us for fifty years so energetically, turn around and testify in front of the Chamber, as the government's representative, in favor of the abolition of the *officiers*?" [28]

In 1891 Brouardel simply reverted to the arguments he had used against the *officiers* in 1873. He again made the point that the *officiers* were not practicing in rural areas as they were intended to and noted that those departments with the poorest distribution of practitioners per inhabitants also had the lowest proportion of *officiers* to *docteurs*. Brouardel also argued that *officiers* were attracted to the cities to an even greater degree than doctors, and were no more eager than doctors to practice in rural areas. Brouardel further claimed that doctors were more likely than *officiers* to establish practice in poor areas and that the statistics on distribution showed that "once again the spirit of sacrifice improves with the degree of education." [29] Brouardel apparently forgot his own previous point that *officiers* did not practice in many poor departments simply because they were prevented from doing so by the regulations governing their practice. After 1891, Brouardel argued that the reason the *officiers* were concentrated in the north of the country was because that was the wealthiest part of the nation. In 1888 he had pointed out that *officiers* were concentrated in the north because this was an area of rapidly growing population which had successfully solved its medical care problems by promoting local medical schools and the training of *officiers*. [30] This in fact was clearly true in the Nord and the Pas-de-Calais (see below).

It is not clear why Brouardel vacillated on the *officiers de santé*. His five years of support for the second order of physicians may be explained by the pressure brought on him by the other members of the

C.C.H.P. for whom the lack of practitioners in many areas of France was the most crucial medical issue of the time. However, it should be pointed that during this time Brouardel's defense of the *officiers* was quite outspoken, strongly argued and well reasoned. His point about the reasons for the geographic concentration of the officiate in the North was a just counter to his earlier complaints about the lack of *officiers* in poorly medicalized departments. Brouardel's only defense of his second change of view on the *officiers,* in contrast, was rather weak. Ignoring medical care issues altogether, Brouardel argued that the 1889 Military Law had changed regulations on the officiate in such a way as to make it far less attractive as a career. The Military Law did away with previous exemptions from military service allowed the *officiers de santé.* It further relegated the *officiers de santé,* once the backbone of the military medical corps, to the lower echelons of the officer corps. In Brouardel's eyes this change would greatly reduce recruits to the *officiers de santé.* [31]

Between 1886 and 1890 the Union conducted a relentless campaign against the officiate. Of course, in direct contrast to the C.C.H.P., the Union felt that there were not too few but too many practitioners in France. The Union doctors were distressed to see the opposite view expressed by the C.C.H.P. and in the popular press. The Union's point of view was based upon considerations other than the distribution of practitioners or the medical needs of the nation. It was based upon the simple principle that as things stood, French doctors allegedly could not make a living in the areas which did not have practitioners. Although they readily admitted that *officiers* had lower financial expectations and more adaptability to rural areas, the Union leaders denied the usefulness of allowing them to continue in practice. [32] The Union's opposition to the officiate was based on the fact that the second grade of practitioners too often competed directly with doctors for clients. In 1889, in a direct attack on Brouardel and the C.C.H.P., the Union adopted Brouardel's 1873 line of argument, claiming that the *officiers* were not filling the role of practitioner in areas which would otherwise be without them, but were instead contributing to the oversupply of practitioners in urban areas. As Brouardel had done in 1873, the Union based this point on a comparison of the distribution of practitioners among the departments. The Union said that Brouardel's 1888 argument that 30,373 communes did not have resident practitioners was absurd because probably none of these communes could actually support a practitioner, either a *docteur* or *officier*. [33]

In explaining Brouardel's change of heart, Cézilly claimed that the president of the C.C.H.P. was persuaded by new statistics which showed that those published by the C.C.H.P. in 1886 were erroneous. [34] However, in reality the new data did not refute the C.C.H.P. statistics; the new data continued to show that about two thousand communes were dependent upon *officiers* as the only available licensed medical care in their area. Further, thirteen departments had suffered a significant loss of *officiers* with no corresponding increase in *docteurs* between 1866 and 1881. These thirteen departments continued to see a decline in the overall number of practitioners and a decline in the ratio of practitioners per population through 1896 (see Table III-1). Brouardel was apparently pursuaded by the Union's intense pressure in favor of a unified profession and the abolition of the officiate. After 1890 Brouardel completely ignored the well reasoned argument he and the C.C.H.P. had been making between 1886 and 1890 in favor of the continuation and expansion of the officiate. [35] The consequences of this was that the legislature never heard the C.C.H.P.'s argument in defense of the *officiers*, for Brouardel was the only member of the C.C.H.P. who spoke in the debates on the legislation. With the prestige of his medical positions, and his position as government representative in the Chamber debates over the law, Brouardel's opposition to the *officiers de santé* carried a great deal of influence with the legislature.

In the legislature the issue of the officiate was debated at length. However, the Chamber was ultimately pursuaded by Brouardel's and Chevandier's argument that the officiate was not fulfilling the role envisioned for it in 1803 as the corps of rural practitioners. But even more powerful was Chevandier's argument that having two orders of practitioners was "anti-democratic." He noted,

"there is in fact only one order of patient; it will not do to have two categories of doctors. The equality of the patient in front of science is a democratic right that the Republic must recognize." [36]

Chevandier went on to argue that the best way of assuring rural medical care was to pass the other provisions of the law on the practice of medicine which would aid physicians in the collections of fees and protect them against unlicensed practitioners. [37] Chevandier also argued that the legislature should pass the law on medical assistance as a way of encouraging doctors to practice in rural areas, and thus counteract any damage to the supply of practitioners that the abolition of the *officiers* might cause.

The opposition to the abolition of the *officiers de santé* was stronger in the Senate than in the Chamber. Rural senators feared the effects of this move on medical care in the countryside. The senators demanded what had not as yet been done by any of the medical authorities, a survey of departmental authorities for their opinion on the issue. The Senate appointed a special committee headed by Union sympathizer, Senator-Dr. Andre Victor Cornil, to carry out the survey. Initially the committee was split on the issue: of eight members, four advocated maintaining the officiate, three were for abolition, and one, Dr. Emile Combes, advocated creating a new kind of second grade of practitioner. [38] Combes, a radical politician who was eventually to preside as premier over the separation of church and state in 1905, was otherwise an ardent supporter of the goals of the doctors' Union movement. Eventually, the opinion of the commission was swayed in favor of abolition as the result of Cornil's survey. Cornil and Gassot prepared the ground in advance for this survey by advising all local syndicats to lobby their departmental council directly in opposition to the officiate. The Union provided its local syndicats with statistics and arguments in favor of the abolition of the *officiers,* to be used in front of the local departmental councils. [39] Of course no counter arguments were given to the departmental councillors.

Cornil reported that the majority of the departments supported the abolition of the officiate. Upon close examination of the reports sent back to Cornil, however, there were some important exceptions. For example, the council of Haute-Vienne agreed to the abolition of the officiate only upon the condition that the departmental medical schools be given a greater role in medical education so that students could do all their course work and take most of their examinations there. The Haute-Vienne council also demanded that more scholarships be made available, and that students be allowed more opportunities to take their examinations. In Meurthe-et-Moselle, the departmental council voted unanimously to maintain the *officiers de santé*. The council noted that although there were few *officiers* still practicing in the department, there were many in nearby Pas-de-Calais. The council felt that the abolition would set back medical care in Pas-de-Calais, and in rural France in general. [40]

In Pas-de-Calais itself, the departmental council was strongly against the abolition of the *officiers*. The councillors felt that they had very good medical care in their department precisely because of the many *officiers de santé*. There were 254 *officiers* practicing in Pas-de-Calais in 1890-91. [41] The council reported that in cases of emergencies, practitioners arrived very quickly and that their effective medical services for indigents was mostly staffed by *officiers*. This medical assistance program was the result of decisions taken in the department in the 1850s to increase the number of *officiers* and use them to establish free medical services. Thus in 1855 the department had enlarged the medical school at Arras to educate more *officiers de santé*.

In neighboring Nord, where there were also a large number of *officiers de santé*, the council likewise voted against the abolition of the officiate. Here the council argued that the *officiers* were capable practitioners who provided good, inexpensive care to rural people. The support given the *officers* in Nord and Pas-de-Calais justified an observation made by Brouardel and members the C.C.H.P. in 1886-88, that in areas of the North which had undergone rapid industrialization and population growth in the latter half of the century, it was the *officiers* who had met the increased needs for medical practitioners. The views of the departmental councils in Nord and Pas-de-Calais were shared by the council of the Somme. [42] Most of the *officiers* in the nation were located in Nord, Pas-de-Calais, Somme and Aisne. Thus in these four departments which both trained and utilized the most *officiers,* three of four strongly opposed their abolition. [43] In the rest of the nation, there were relatively few *officiers* and thus it was not at all surprising that most of their councils would be convinced that the second grade of practitioners was dying out anyway and might as well be abolished.

In several other departments with large and relatively poor rural populations, the councils also voted against the abolition of the *officiers,* for fear of exacerbating their already serious lack of licensed practitioners. These departments included Puy-de-Dôme, Seine-Inférieure, Calvados, and Hautes-Pyrenées. [44] In Haute-Vienne, the council agreed to the abolition of the *officiers* but on the condition that a new second grade of *docteurs* be created which would have the same titles and capabilities as

the first grade of *docteurs,* but with less lengthy educational requirements. [45] In Seine-Inférieure, an anonymous defender of the medical
school at Rouen complained than the abolition of the officiate would
make medical education even more centralized in Paris that it already
was. This writer believed that practitioners trained locally were more
apt to stay in practice locally. Further, he argued that the training they
received at Rouen was superior to that received in Paris in several
respects. Also he said that in their clinical training, students had more
direct contact with patients in the provincial schools and their attached
hospitals. In the provinces students did not develop the conceits of the
Paris elites, and thus retained a humble character more sympathetic to
the poor, rural sick. [46] A Doctor from Calvados shared the feelings of
the writer from Seine-Inférieure. He also felt that conditions in the
countryside were such that *docteurs,* having spent many years and great
expense on their baccalaureate and medical training at the faculties,
would not have the temperament to practice in the countryside where
they could not hope to earn over three thousand francs a year. The
officiers de santé, he felt, had more patience and lower expectation than
young *docteurs* and could thus better cope with the difficult conditions
of the rural areas. [47]

These objections to the abolition of the officiate and the connected
concerns over availability of practitioners were largely ignored in the
legislature and the medical press. Cornil simply reported that the
majority of departments supported the abolition of the *officiers.* Cornil
did not mention the fact that in those departments which utilized a large

number of *officiers,* the councils opposed their abolition. He briefly mentioned that there was concern that the countryside not be deprived of practitioners but implied that some slight changes in the educational requirements would solve this problem and satisfy the departments. Jules de Crisenoy of the C.S.A.P. (Conseil supérieur de l'Assistance publique), noted that many departments which had voted in favor of the abolition of the *officiers* did so on the condition that educational changes be made so that medical training was more accessible to a wider sector of the population. Specifically, many departmental councils advocated doing away with the study of Latin and Greek as requirements for valid secondary degrees and wanted to see the creation of more scholarships to the faculties and medical schools. Crisenoy suported these changes but also noted that they were precisely what the Union movement wished to avoid. [48] The legislature had already decided that educational requirements would not be outlined by the law on the practice of medicine, but would be left up to the Ministry of Education to establish by decree. [49] The legislative committee on the law, headed by Chevandier, placated the representatives of the provincial medical schools by assuring them that planned changes from the Ministry of Education would increase their role in the training of *docteurs.* [50] When these medical schools were brought around to abolition by Chevandier's promises, the officiate lost an important source of support.

The other major issue of debate over the Loi Chevandier was the unionization of physicians. Article Thirteen of the law extended to physicians the rights given to other occupational groups in 1884. [51] There was some opposition to this article in the Chamber, but the main challenge arose when the article was discussed in the Senate in March 1892. Between the law's hearing in the Chamber and Senate, a new cabinet came into power under the moderate, Emile Loubet. Loubet took the Ministry of Interior as well as the presidency of the Council of Ministers. As Minister of Interior he supported the objections to the article raised by Henri Monod and members of the C.C.H.P. and C.S.A.P. Monod and Loubet feared that giving physicians the right to strike would jeopardize the projected medical assistance program. Loubet argued that although doctors had legitimate interests to defend, their relationship to the state was more complicated than that of other professions. In addition to their private practice, many of them occupied bureaucratic positions as well both on the national and local levels of government. Moreover, Loubet maintained that current programs called for doctors to be allied to the state more closely than ever. He further pointed out that the version drafted by the C.C.H.P. had not contained an article legalizing physicians' syndicats, even though it was well known in the committee that this was what doctors desired. Loubet and Monod feared that if given the right to strike, physicians would use it against state programs. [52] Cézilly called this fear "illusory;" however, subsequent events in the application of the Medical Assistance Law proved that the fears of Loubet and Monod were justified. [53]

The most outspoken opponents of Article Thirteen in the Senate were conservative senators known for their opposition to the separation of church and state, such as Senator Louis Buffet, René Marie Herve de Saisy, and the Marquis de l'Angle Beaumanoir. [54] Conservative Senator Herve de Saisy was the greatest enemy of the Union movement in the Senate. He sarcastically proposed to amend the Loi Chevandier so that anyone *other than* doctors and *officier de santé* could practice medicine. [55] Some senators felt that the doctors syndicats would not operate in the best interests of patients. Some conservatives pointed out that that since it was impossible for patients to unionize, doctors should not be able to either. Further, they feared that doctors would simply use their syndicats as a way of raising their fees. The opposing senators also argued that many doctors were in effect *fonctionnaires,* and therefore should not have the right to strike. [56] It was not only conservatives who opposed Article Thirteen; left-republican Senator Henri Louis Tolain, who introduced the 1884 law on syndicats in the Senate, was also opposed to syndicalization for physicians. Much to the dismay of *Le Concours,* he argued that the syndicat law was aimed at benefiting workers, not bourgeois professionals. Another Left-Republican, Senator Louis Goblet, noted for his insistence on de-centralization and his defense of the prerogatives of the communes, also opposed Article Thirteen on the grounds that it interfered too much in local affairs. [57]

In response to the Senate's rejection of Article Thirteen, *Le Concours* unleashed a frenzied defense of unionization. The society and Union leaders claimed that the syndicats were not intended to be used against individual patients or government authorities. In truth the syndi-cats had advocated their right to strike against non-paying clients; this was to be achieved through the creation of the "black books," lists of patients who were to avoided by doctors because of their not paying medical bills (See Chapter I). [58] By 1892, the Union movement had abandoned this project, but still demanded the right to refuse service to the clients of insurance societies against which they had grievances. In fact numerous strikes of this kind were undertaken by local societies in the period 1880-1914. [59] The Union movement had also given its sup-port to a strike of German doctors against the City of Tilsit just four months before the Loi Chevandier was discussed in the Senate. [60] *Le Concours* did not hesitate to bargain professional goals for bureaucratic ones. In a veiled threat to Monod, Cézilly stated that if the government expected the cooperation of doctors in their plans for the creation of public health and medical assistance programs, they would have to meet the demands of private practitioners. [61] The members of *Le Concours* also loudly complained that the opposition of many senators resulted from the general hostility of French society against doctors. Gassot decried the animosity directed toward doctors in the Senate and com-plained that for many senators, doctors were pariahs. [62]

Several prestigious voices lead the defense of the Union movement in the Senate: Senators Cornil, Combes, and Ludovic Trarieux. Trarieux was a left-republican, noted, like Combes for his anti-Boulangist, pro-laicization politics. Cornil was a moderate who presented the Loi Chevandier as well as the Medical Assistance Law to the Senate. [63] These senators defended the right of doctors to organize on the grounds which the Union movement had been emphasizing since its founding. Cornil pointed out that in effect patients were unionizing against doctors by joining insurance societies. Further, he argued that under the Union movement, local syndicats were the best way of combating the illegal practice of medicine. As a group, doctors could gather the kind of funds and legal expertise necessary to prosecute illegal practitioners in the courts, and the articles of the Loi Chevandier on illegal practice explicitly gave the syndicats the right to bring legal action against illegal practitioners. [64]

To make Article Thirteen more acceptable to the Senate, Cornil worked out an amendment. The amendment was the result of a compromise between Cornil, Monod and Loubet. Cornil and Loubet realized that the main issue was to draft the article in such a way that the public health and public assistance bureaucrats would not feel that their programs were threatened. The solution was to stipulate that doctors could not organize against the state; thus it was understood that doctors would be prevented from striking against the state, departments or communes. Brouardel reported that Loubet's intervention was crucial; once he was satisfied by the protestations of Cézilly and Fourmestreaux and the assurances of Brouardel that the syndicats would not organize against the state, the Senate changed its mind. Loubet returned to the Senate in April to assure that body that doctors only wanted to organize to provide assistance to one another, establish friendly ties and prosecute illegal practitioners. [65]

To help convince the senators of the Union's benign intentions, Cornil read a letter from Fourmestreaux and Cézilly in which the Union leaders denied any intent to organize against governemnt authorities or patients. The doctors' only enemies, they claimed, were illegal practitioners and insurance societies. Meanwhile, the Union leadership hastily organized a program to contact senators directly to lobby in favor of syndicalization. [66] As a result of the assurances of Cornil, Loubet and the Union, the amended Article Thirteen was narrowly passed by the Senate in April 1892. Ironically, exactly what Monod feared happened. The legalized doctors syndicats had a tremendous impact on the implementation of the Medical Assistance Law after it was enacted in 1893. Supported by the Union, numerous local syndicats did strike against departmental medical assistance programs between 1893 and 1902. During these developments the amendment to Article Thirteen was largely ignored. [67]

Besides these two major points, the Loi Chevandier contained several other important changes which the Union movement counted on to improve the economic and social conditions of physicians in private practice. There were two general forms to these changes: articles which helped in the collection of fees and articles which helped to eliminate competition.

The further elimination of competition was achieved through stronger penalties against illegal practice and greater restrictions on the practice of the other legal medical practitioners. Some of these restrictions again created conflict between the Union on one hand and the

C.C.H.P. and the some members of the Chamber and Senate on the other. Principally these conflicts centered on the practice of midwives. The original Chevandier version of the law prohibited dentists and midwives from using anesthetics or prescribing medicine. The C.C.H.P. argued that dentists should be allowed to use local anesthetics and this position was supported by the Chamber. [68] The final version of the law, however, retained these restrictions against midwives. Since the late eighteenth century, French midwives were required to be licensed and to undergo a specific training course. [69] Dentists, however, had no such requirements to guarantee their expertise, although in the 1890s the educational ministry was in the process of writing licensing requirements for them. Thus it was not for reasons of technical ability that the legislature granted the use of anesthetics to dentists while denying it to midwives. Perhaps the legislature was more concerned about toothaches than labor pains. Certainly the licensed midwives, who were move numerous than doctors in 1891, consituted a major competitive threat to doctors who had been trying for several decades to establish their dominance in obstetrics and gynecology. [70] While the C.C.H.P. was silent on the prohibitions of the *Loi Chavandier* against the use of anesthetics by midwives, it did take some actions in the midwives' favor. At the time that the law was being discussed in legislature, the committee issued a decree which allowed midwives to purchase certain previously restricted substances used for antiseptic and anesthetic purposes. [71]

Midwives were also defended by conservatives in the Senate. In the version of the law passed by the Chamber, the second grade of midwives had been eliminated. The second grade of midwives was licensed by departmental authorities while the first order of midwives was licensed through examination at the faculties of medicine or at provincial schools of medicine. This second grade license was very common in the more remote areas of the country, far from medical schools and faculties. A group of conservative senators from rural constituencies argued that the medical care in their areas had already suffered enough from the abolition of the officiate. They convinced the Senate, and ultimately the Chamber as well, to preserve the second order of midwives in the *Loi Chevandier*. [72]

In addition to restrictions on the practice of midwives and dentists, the law contained harsher regulations on the illegal practice of medicine. The 1803 law on the practice of medicine had prescribed maximum penalties of fifteen francs, with no prison sentences required upon conviction for the illegal practice of medicine. Physicians complained that these penalties were so light that illegal practitioners who were prosecuted under the 1803 law were not discouraged from returning to their illegal occupation and in fact benefited from the publicity that an arrest entailed. [73] The Loi Chevandier prescribed much greater penalties for illegal practice: a minimum of one hundred and a maximum of five hundred francs. In the case of repeated offenses, the fine was doubled and the guilty party was to be imprisoned for fifteen days to six months. Under the Loi Chevandier the illegal practice of dentistry or midwifery carried fines of fifty to one hundred francs, and in the case of recidivism the fine was doubled and the criminal was to be imprisoned. An additional crime was defined by the Loi Chevandier, the usurption of the title of *docteur* or *officier de santé,* for which fine was one to two thousand francs; in the case of recidivism, the fine was two to three thousand francs and a mandatory prison sentence of three months to a year. For the usurption of the title of midwife, the fine under the Loi Chevandier was one hundred to five thousand frances and a prison sentence of six to fifteen days in the case of a repeat offense. The law also made it illegal for anyone to use the title doctor in conjunction with his name without a degree awarded in France, unless the place of origin of the degree was also indicated. This article of the law was aimed specifically at the degrees which many illegal practitioners were obtaining by mail from the United States. [74]

The Union movement had hoped to change the definition of illegal practice in such a way as to make it easier to prosecute certain kinds of non-licensed practitioners. Private physicians in the syndicats believed that they lost many clients to priests and nuns, and even to school teachers. They accused these authority figures of giving medical advice which amounted to consultations. Thus in the original version of the law proposed by Chevandier, the definition of illegal practice included "habitual consultation." However, the Chamber refused to support this on the grounds that it was customary for people to discuss medical issues and seek informal advice. Instead they suggested the phrase "directions followed." The entire sentence was worded in such a away as to be rather vague but the impression was left that illegal practice had to involve actual treatments of some kind. [75] In spite of this modification, the total effect of the new regulations on illegal practice, coupled with the new ability of the doctors to prosecute illegals through their syndicats, meant that the Loi Chevandier gave doctors far greater weapons against illegal practitioners than they had ever possessed before. Certainly, as reflected in *Le Concours* and the other publications of the Union and syndicats, the period beween 1892 and 1902 was marked by great syndicat activity in publicizing and prosecuting illegal practitioners. [76]

In addition to the regulations on illegal practice, the Loi Chevandier also made certain reforms in the Civil Code which helped doctors in the collection of fees. These reforms were seen by the Union as very important in improving the economic position of doctors and promoting their self-respect. Under article 2272 of the Civil Code physicians had one year in which to sue clients for fees. Doctors argued that this time limit was too short. In the Chevandier version the Civil Code was to be amended to increase the time limit to five years. The Chamber passed this article but the Senate reduced the limit to two years. This change was advocated by Dr. F. de Ranse of the influential *Gazette médicale de Paris,* who believed it was too cruel for clients and particularly the heirs of a dead client to have the threat of a doctor's suit hanging over their head for five years. [77] The Loi Chevandier also extended the right of doctors to claim creditors' prerogatives upon the death of a client who owed medical bills. Previously article 2101 of the Civil Code had usually been construed in such a way that doctors could only claim creditors' prerogatives for fees involved in the treatment of the illness leading directly to the death of the client. The Loi Chevandier amended the article to extend this right to include any illness regardless of the outcome. [78]

Besides the *officier de santé,* the other major issue of disagreement between the C.C.H.P. and the Chevandier versions of the law on the practice of medicine dealt with the declaration of cases of epidemic disease. As we have seen, the C.C.H.P. held such declaration to be crucial to the monitoring and control of disease. The Chevandier version of the law contained a very vague article on the responsibilites of private physicians who came into contact with cases of contagious disease. This article stipulated that

"All doctors are held responsible to furnish to administrative authorities or health officials information useful to maintaining public health, especially regarding epidemic or endemic diseases and cause of death, under the reserve of professional secrecy." [79]

On this point the C.C.H.P. version was far more specific; it read:

"All doctors, *officier de santé* and midwives are held responsible, under penalties prescribed in article 27 of the present law, to make known to public authorities within twenty-four hours any case of contagious disease which comes to their attention. A list of these diseases will be prepared by the Ministry of Interior, with the advice of the Academy of Medicine and the Public Health Committee. An administrative regulation will fix the manner in which the declaration of these diseases will be made." [80]

The C.C.H.P. noted that such requirements had already been written into the public health regulations of Great Britain and the City of New York. [81] Moreover, since 1881 the French state had required the declaration of cases of contagious disease among animals. The committee argued that the nation owed as much protection to its humans as it provided to its animals. [82] The committee further argued that this regulation was only a first step toward organizing a comprehensive service to gather accurate statistics on disease and cause of death in the entire nation. They planned to model this program after that which had been instituted in the city of Paris by the Paris Statistics Committee under the leadership of Louis Adolphe Bertillon. This idea was supported by the Academy of Medicine, the Société de médecine publique et d'hygiène professionnelle, the A.G.M.F., as well as by Brouardel, Monod, A.J. Martin and all of France's important hygienists. [83] However, it was not supported by private doctors or the syndicat movement. The idea of declaration was strongly protested by the syndicat movement and also by the editors of several of the most prestigious medical journals. [84]

There were several things in the C.C.H.P. version of the article on declaration which private doctors found objectionable. The C.C.H.P. made the obligation to declare cases of contagious disease much more specific, and, further, put the public health bureaucracy in a position of telling doctors what diseases would be subject to declaration and how the declaration would be made. Under the C.C.H.P. version, the declaration of contagious disease would become a regularized procedure. Most objectionable to doctors was the idea that they would be subject to penalties if they did not comply. The idea of declaring contagious diseases to public authorities elicited tremendous discussion and protest from private physicians. They found the idea repugnant and threatening.

Private physicians argued that the requirement to declare cases of contagious disease was a violation of professional secrecy, enshrined by article 378 of the Civil Code. The C.C.H.P. argued that while some medical situations called for professional confidentiality, many did not. Brouardel and Martin held that secrecy was required in the case of venereal disease, diseases thought to be hereditary, injuries received under delicate circumstances such as during an insurrection, a duel, or at a brothel. They also felt that the patient's prognosis should be kept confidential. Brouardel thought it appropriate to keep certain diagnoses from the patient himself, especially in cases of tuberculosis and heart disease, in order not to spoil the life these people had left. [85] In cases other than these, the C.C.H.P. felt a declaration of public authorities did not violate professional secrecy.

Private physicians felt otherwise. They resented any interference of public authorities in their relationships with their clients, which they characterized as based on the utmost trust and discretion. As G. Drouineau envisioned him, the physician was in a special position of trust as the intimate confidant of the family, in possession of information about all of their moral as well as physical dilemmas. [86] On a more practical level, physicians claimed that they risked losing clients if it was known that the presence of contagious disease in a home or business would not be kept secret. Physicians noted that it was a matter of family pride and reputation that such things be kept confidential, and in the case of hereditary disease it was necessary to be discreet in order not to spoil the children's matrimonial chances. [87] However, the most serious objections were economic; doctors explained that shopkeepers feared that if it was known in an area that there was disease in or near a shop or restaurant, the customers would disappear. Cézilly said frankly that such a situation put a doctor between "...his duty and his interest." [88] Although public authorities were also supposed to guard confidentiality, physicians' claimed they did not trust them to do so. [89] Moreover, physicians complained that the responsibility of declaration was an unwarranted nuisance and a waste of the doctor's valuable time. [90]

The C.C.H.P. and the Union worked out a compromise on the declaration article. Under the compromise, officially proposed by Brouardel, the head of the family was made primarily responsible for reporting the disease and the doctor was charged to report only if the family head refused to do so. Both the family head and doctor were subject to fines if they did not comply with their respective duties. [91] Many doctors continued to complain about this new version, feeling that authorities in practice would be far more likely to hold doctors responsible than family fathers. Cézilly, however, seems to have acquiesced as a trade-off for Brouardel's support on Article Thirteen which legalized the unionization of doctors. At the time of the debate over Article Thirteen, Cézilly stated that the public health authorities should support the

Union on that issue if they expected the movement to support them on the public health aspects of the law. [92] Ultimately, the compromise had no effect as the Senate refused to accept the idea of holding grieving relatives responsible for reporting the cause of the death of a family member. [93] They returned to the original C.C.H.P. version, which was also in turn accepted by Chamber on reconsideration. [94] Physicians felt they had been betrayed by the C.C.H.P. It should also be pointed out that the opposition to holding doctors responsible for declaration was not confined to private practitioners. In spite of the official support for declaration given by the A.G.M.F. and the Academy of Medicine, some eminent names in medicine objected. Dr. F. de Ranse, editor of the *Gazette médicale de Paris,* expressed the hope that the provisions of the Loi Chevandier requiring declaration would be ignored by doctors. [95]

The passage of the Loi Chevandier was followed by a decree from Henri Monod which listed the contagious diseases subject to declaration. The list was prepared by the Academy of Medicine and the C.C.H.P.; it included typhus, smallpox, scarlet fever, diphtheria, military fever, cholera, plague, yellow fever, dysentery, puerperal fever, and eye infections of newborns. The list clearly conformed to Martin and Brouardel's notion of what conditions should not be reported, but was still too extensive for most doctors. [96]

Lack of compliance was widespread, as doctors continued to interpret the article on professional secrecy in the civil code in the broadest possible way. In 1900 the C.C.H.P. reported that in only seventy-five of 350 arrondissements was the declaration of contagious disease being done in a satisfactory manner. [97] The committee continued to urge declaration upon doctors but in spite of requirements and penalties in two laws, they did not support the prosecution of doctors for failing to report diseases on the list. Brouardel said that it was not unexpected that it would be difficult to get the medical profession to alter its old habits, but chided doctors for forgetting that their first obligation was to the overall health of the population. [98] The physicians' view, however, was that their first obligation was to the patient and family. Doctors also gave other reasons for their opposition to declaration, claiming that mayors and other local officials sometimes pressured doctors to protect their town's reputation. An incident in Arpajon in 1895 illustrates this problem. A doctor sent a declaration of five cases of diphtheria to the mayor only to have an article appear in the "Echo arpajonnais" criticizing him for trying to cause needless alarm. The local newspaper claimed that the disease was not diphtheria, but only laryngitis. The doctor sucessfully prosecuted the mayor's secretary in court for not keeping the declaration confidential. [99] Doctors also pointed out that in rural areas the declaration of contagious disease served no purpose because there were no services or funds for disinfection or anti-contagion measures. Moreover local residents were often very uncooperative in efforts to isolate patients, refusing to close businesses and insisting on making visits to the rooms and homes of the afflicted. [100]

Doctors particularly objected to puerperal fever (childbed fever) being included on the list. It was widely known by the 1890s that this affliction was often transmitted through the agency of doctors and midwives attending births. It was therefore particularly embarrassing for a physician to have to report a case among his clientele because it would reflect badly on his own attention to hygiene. Thus physicians argued that puerperal fever should never be reported because such a disclosure also indicated, of course, that the patient was pregnant and pregnancy should always be kept confidential. It is interesting that they did not make this objection with regard to the declaration of eye infections in newborn infants, even though such information would also of course reveal a pregnancy! Monod reacted to this position by arguing that the disclosure of puerperal fever was quite important for the control of the infection and the identification of those responsible for its transmission. He eventually stipulated that peurperal fever only fell under professional secrecy if the client had made it clear that she intended to keep her pregnancy secret. [101]

The Union movement complained loudly against declaration again while the Public Health Law was being discussed. They feared, apparently, that this law might see the real enforcement of declaration, as C.C.H.P. officials hoped it would. The Union leadership felt it had been betrayed by Brouardel as well as by Senators Cornil and Leon Labbé, all of whom worked to back an article on declaration in the Public Health Law. [102] By the time that the Public Health Law was passed in 1902, the greatest concerns of doctors and public health officials involved the declaration of tuberculosis. As discussed in the last chapter, the Permanent Anti-Tuberculosis Committee was involved in a controversy over the accuracy of tuberculosis statistics. A large part of the problem, the committee believed, was caused by the reluctance of doctors to risk the patronage of the families they served by revealing cases of this socially sensitive illness. [103] The Union movement was greatly angered to note that in 1901, at the same time that the Public Health Law was being considered, the tuberculosis committee, the C.C.H.P., and the Academy of Medicine were calling for the inclusion of tuberculosis on the list of diseases subject to declaration. The Union stated its intention to "bring some sense" into the practice of declaration, which meant, essentially, supporting doctors who ignored it. [104] In the years immediately after the passage of the 1902 Public Health Law, Henri Monod and other hygienists continued to complain that doctors were very uncooperative in reporting cases of contagious disease. [105]

While the Union movement was forced to accept some modifications of the new regulations it wanted on the practice of medicine, the Loi Chevandier must be seen as a great Union victory. Through this law private physicians achieved several goals they had greatly desired since at least the 1840s: the abolition of the *officiers de santé,* further limitations on the practice of midwives, greater restrictions against illegal practice, as well as a more recent goal, the legalization of their Union movement. These provisions gave them a firm monopoly over the practice of medicine, something they had long desired.

It is crucial to note that the Loi Chevandier did not originate in the Academy of Medicine, the Ministry of Education (as in the 1840s) or the A.G.M.F., but in the Union movement. Thus the law represents the arrival of private practitioners as leaders of their own profession and as powerful arbitrators of the medical care system. The Loi Chevandier was a law by and for private practitioners and it enshrined medical practice on their terms. Medicine would be dominated by a group, originating in one social class and undergoing the same education and socialization process, determined to protect and promote a rigid view of how medical care would be applied. This view emphasized medical care as a private, one-to-one encounter between physician and client with a minimum of bureaucratic or institutional interference. Moreover it would be left completely up to the profession to determine the rules and costs governing the application of their expertise. Through their syndicats the profession would control illegal practice, fees, clienteles, and relationships between practitioners. The Union movement would also give individual practioners support in resisting the demands of the public health bureaucracy.

It has been frequently noted in the histories of the Third Republic that physicians were a strong backbone of republican politics. What has not been considered was how this political influence was brought to bear on medical issues and medical legislation. It is clear that the corps of doctors in the Chamber and Senate were of major importance in the achievement of the Loi Chevandier. However, the Union movement itself must also be given considerable credit. The Union noted the climate of the times: the solidarist ideology with its concern with protecting the population and integrating all parts of society into the Republic. The doctors successfully appealed to the legislature on these very grounds. Portraying themselves as hygienists, the doctors of the Union movemnt sold themselves and private practice as the agents of the bacteriological revolution. In addition, the Union used the argument of democracy to convince the legislature that equality in medical care meant all citizens should have access to the same sort of practitioners: physicians, and no others, arguing that to have different practitioners for urban and rural populations would be "undemocratic." Further, the Union effectively used the improved public image of medicine as well as populationist concerns to argue that the Loi Chevandier would help spread information about the new scientific discoveries and help the population problem. In fact, there was no evidence that doctors alone could have much effect on the national health. It was the public health measures that could, and eventually would, make a positive impact on mortality. But private physicians were successful in the legislature in 1893-94 while hygienists largely failed. The complete success of this medical legislative program must be attributed in no small part to this dynamic Union movement which incorporated the professional desires of the private practitioners and adapted their rhetoric to the goals of solidarism.

The story behind the Loi Chevandier also demonstrates how solidarist ideology, aimed at piecemeal social reform, was able to unite republican politicians who normally disagreed on other issues. Radicals such Combes and Trarieaux united with moderates and progressists like Chevandier and Cornil to get the law through the Chamber and Senate. This unity was responsible for other solidarist legislation such as the 1894 law on low-cost housing and the 1893 law on medical assistance. Republicans could not agree on religious issues but could come together on legislation which was presented as preserving the population and combating class divisions by bringing all the classes the benefits of modernization and thus incorporating them into the republican synthesis.

TABLE III-I

DEPARTMENTS WITH GREATEST LOSS OF OFFICIER DE SANTE
1866-1896(1)

	OFFICIERS DE SANTE		PERCENT CHANGE	TOTAL PRACTI- TIONERS		PERCENT CHANGE	DISTRIBUTION OF TOTAL PRACTITION- ERS. ONE PER-		PERCENT CHANGE
	1866	1896		1866	1896		1866	1896	
AISNE	125	44	-65	227	189	-17	2487	2867	-15
AUBE	79	4	-94	157	97	-38	1694	2649	-56
COTES-DU-NORD	74	20	-73	145	105	-28	4337	5867	-35
GERS	186	47	-75	313	172	-45	955	1639	-72
ILLE-ET-VILAINE	118	68	-42	197	204	+04	2969	3049	-03
LANDES	115	34	-70	211	160	-25	1425	1887	-33
MARNE	103	35	-66	207	182	-12	1862	2415	-30
NORD	261	162	-38	464	613	+32	2809	2956	-05
PAS-DE-CALAIS	226	126	-44	323	268	-17	2243	3386	-50
HAUTES-PYRÉNÉES	122	41	-66	196	97	-50	1225	1598	-30
PYRÉNÉES-ORIENTALES	104	29	-72	164	187	+14	1109	2193	-97
SOMME	216	123	-43	305	120	-27	1877	2573	-37
CALVADOS	95	30	-68	243	144	-40	1979	3055	-54
AVERAGE CHANGE			-63			-19			-40

1. R.T.C.C.H.P., V. 16 (1886); Dr. Maurice Lesieur, Répertoire officiel
de la Médicine et de la Pharmacie Francais, 1896.

NOTES TO CHAPTER III

1. Dr. F. de Ranse, "Le médecin et la médecine de nos jours," *Gazette médicale de Paris,* Series 7, Vol. VI, N. 14, p 165.

2. Dr. Aymard, "Les premiers effets de l'encombrement," *Bul. des syn. méd de France,* (May 1901), p 1039.

3. *Le Concours,* V. 10, N. 1, (Jan 7, 1888), p 1; V. 15, N. 48, (December 2, 1893), p 567; *Lyon médical,* N. 27, (July 6, 1890).

4. Dr. F. Ranse, *Ibid.*

5. "Assemblée générale de la Société du Concours médical, Oct. 20, 1889," *Bul. des Syn. des méd. de France,* N. 37, (Nov. 1889), pp 317-319.

6. *Ibid.*

7. *Ibid.*

8. *Ibid.*

9. *Ibid.*

10. On November 23, 1889: *Gazette médicale de Paris,* 62nd year, Series 7, V. VIII, N. 14, (April 4, 1891); *Le Courrier médical,* V. 41, N. 5, (Jan 31, 1891), p 49; two other versions of the law were proposed at about the same time, one by Lockroy on November 23, and another

by David on Feburary 20, 1890. The ancien régime of medical practice, which had supported a dual order of doctors and surgeons, was abolished in 1792, at which time the nation experimented with open medical practice. After a great outcry of protest from influential medical doctors, the nation returned to a system of monopoly when the Revolution took its swing to the right.

11. This law was actually passed by the *Chambre des pairs,* but the revolution intervened before it was considered by the *Chambre des députés;* there was also an earlier abortive project put forth by the Academy of Médecine in 1833: *Gazette médicale de Paris,* Series 7, 62nd year, V. VIII, N. 14, (April 4, 1891), pp 157-160.

12. "l'Exercise de la Médecine," *Le Courrier médical,* V. 41, N. 5, (Jan. 31, 1891; R.C.C.H.P., V. 20, (1890), pp 39-55.

13. see Sussman; Léonard, Thèse; and Robert Haller, "Officiers de Santé, the Second Class Doctors of Nineteenth Century France," *Medical History,* V. 22, N. 1, (Jan, 1878), pp 25-43.

14. V. 16, 1886.

15. Léonard, Thèse, 1978; Flaubert, *Madame Bovary.*

16. "Licensed general practitioners" includes *officiers* and *docteurs* and excludes midwives and pharmacists who were also licensed, but had great limitations on their practice: R.C.C.H.P., V. 16, (1886), pp 124-125.

17. Brouardel, Bergeron, Cornil, Grancher, A.J. Martin, Monod, and Proust, among others: R.C.C.H.P., V. 20, (1890), p 39.

18. R.C.C.H.P., V. 3, (1873), pp 377-79.

19. Sussman.

20. R.C.C.H.P., V. 16, (1886) pp 88-89.

21. *Ibid,* pp 90-91.

22. R.C.C.H.P., pp 92-92.

23. Dr. Magitot, "La Loi Chevandier," *Le Concours,* V. 13, N. 36, (Sept, 5, 1891), pp 439-440; Exerpt from *Normandie médicale,* printed in Le Concours, V. 13, N. 23, (June 7, 1890), pp 272-273.

24. *Ibid,* pp 92-93.

25. *Ibid,* pp 96-97.

26. Brouardel, *De l'Exercise et de l'Enseignement de la médecine,* 1873, pp 10-13.

27. Brouardel, "Du maintien des officiers de santé," *Gazette des Hôpitaux,* (Nov. 6, 1888), pp 1173-74.

28. Dr. Magitot, "La Loi Chevandier," reprint from *Le Temps,* printed in Le Concours, V. 13, N. 36, (Sept 5, 1891), pp 439; *Le Concours,* V. 12, N. 23 (June 7, 1890), pp 272-73.

29. *De l'Exercise et de l'Enseignement de la Médecine.*

30. *Ibid;* Brouardel, "Du maintien des officiers de santé," *Ibid.*

31. *Gazette médicale de Paris,* series 7, V. VIII, N. 14, (April 4, 1891), p 160.

32. Dr. A. Barat-Dulaurier, "Encore la question des officiers de santé," *Bul. des Syn. des méd. de Fr.,* N. 33, (1889) pp 265-268.

33. *Ibid.*

34. Cézilly, *Le Concours,* V. 13, N. 36, (Sept 5, 1891), p 439.

35. *Gazette Hebd. des Sciences médicales de Bordeaux,* V. 12, N. 34, (August 23, 1891), p 405; R.C.C.H.P., V. 20, pp 39-55; F. Ranse, *Gazette médicale de Paris,* 62nd year, Series 7, V. VIII, N. 14, (April 4, 1891), pp 157-60.

36. *Journal Officiel, Débats Parlementaires,* N. 75, (March 17, 1891), p 654.

37. *Ibid.*

38. *La France médicale,* V. 39, N. 24, (June 12, 1891), p 382.

39. *Le Concours,* V. 13, N. 36, (Dept 5, 1891).

40. J. de Crisenoy, "Enquête sur la supression de l'Officate," *Questions d'assistance publique traitées dans les conseils généraux,* (hereinafter, Questions), 1891, pp 262-63.

41. *Ibid,* pp 250-56.

42. *Ibid.*

43. Brouardel, "Du maintain des officiers de santé," *Lancette-française, Gazette des Hôpitaux,* N. 127, (Nov. 6, 1888), pp 1173-74; de Crisenoy, *Ibid.* Gironde also had a smaller but significant percentage of *officiers.* No information was available on the opinion of the departmental council of Aisne on the abolition of the *officiate.* Not all of the departments responded to the survey.

44. *Le Concours,* V. 13, N. 44, (Oct. 31 1891) pp 525-526.

45. *Ibid,* pp 257, 260-62.

46. Excerpt from *Normandie médicale,* reprinted in *Le Concours,* V. 12, N. 23, (June 7, 1890), pp 272-74.

47. *Le Concours,* Ibid.

48. Crisenoy, *Ibid.*

49. *Ibid.*

50. *Gazette Hebd. des Sciences médicales de Bordeaux,* Va. 12, N. 34. (August, 1891) p 405.

51. In the draft of the law passed by the Chamber and considered by the Senate, the article legalizing syndicats for physicians was article fourteen. In the final version enacted into law, the article legalizing the syndicats was article 13, due the combination of articles one and two of the original version.

52. Brouardel, *La Profession médicale,* p 94; "Les Syndicats médicaux devant le Sénat," *Le Concours,* V. 14, N. 13, (Mar. 26, 1892).

53. *Le Concours,* V. 14, N. 14, (April 2, 1892). See chapters III and IV.

54. Tristan-Louis, son of Louis-Joseph l'Angle-Beaumanoir: Adolphe Robert, *Dictionnaire des Parlementaires français* 1891.

55. *Le Concours,* V. 14, N. 17, (April 23, 1892), p 193.

56. *Le Concours,* V. 14, N. 15, (April 9, 1892), pp 169-177.

57. *Le Concours,* V. 14, N. 17, (April 23, 1892), p 193.

58. See Chapter I.

59. See chapter V; also see: *Le Concours,* V. 14, N. 31, (July 30, 1892), p 70 and N. 9 (Feb. 27, 1892) p 105.

60. *Le Concours,* V. 14, N. 4, (Jan 23, 1892) p 47.

61. *Le Concours,* V. 14, N. 13, (Mar 26, 1892).

62. *Le Concours,* V. 14, N. 17, (April 23, 1892), p 193.

63. *Ibid; La France médicale,* V. 39, N. 13, Mars. 1893.

64. *Ibid.*

65. Brouardel, *La Profession médicale,* pp 95.

66. *Le Concours,* V. 14, N. 14, (April 2, 1892).

67. See Chapter IV.

68. R.C.C.H.P. V. 16, (1886), pp 113-131; *Journal Officiel, Débats par-lementaires,* N. 76, (March 19, 1891), pp 658-661.

69. Jacques Gélis, "Sage-femmes et accoucheurs," *AESC,* (Sept-Oct, 1977) V. 32, N. 5.

70. *Ibid.*

71. R.C.C.H.P., V. 16, (1886), pp 97-99; V. 20, (1890), pp 113-117; V. 3 (1874), pp 383-4. see also *Gazette médicale de Paris,* Series 7, V. VIII, N. 17, (April 25, 1891), p 196.

72. R.C.C.H.P., V. 16 (1886), pp 113-121; *Journal Officiel, Débats par-'ementaires,* N. 77 (March 20, 1892) p 674-75; Senator Paul Bourgeois also spoke out in defense of the second order of midwives.

73. *Gazette médicale de Paris,* Series 7, V. VIII, N. 27 (July 4, 1891), pp 316-318;

74. *Gazette médicale de Paris,* Series 7, V. VIII, N. 21 (May 23, 1891), pp 316-318; *Gazette médicale de Paris,* Series 7, V. VIII, N. 29 (July 18, 1891), pp 431-343.

75. *Gazette médicale de Paris,* Series 7, V. VIII, N. 27, (July 4, 1891), pp 316-320.

76. *La Fédération médicale,* see issues from 1902-03; *Le Concours,* V. 14, N. 12, (Mar. 19, 1892), p 143; *Bul. Off. de l'Union des méd. de Fr.,* issues from 1895-1902.

77. *Gazette médicale de Paris,* Series 7, V. VIII, N. 21, (May 23, 1891), pp 345-56.

78. *Ibid.*

79. R.C.C.H.P., v. 20, (1890), p 51.

80. *Ibid.*

81. In Great Britain, both the head of the family and the doctors were held responsible to make declaration to public authorities. In New York, only the physician was held responsible: *Ibid.*

82. R.C.C.H.P., V. 23, (1893), p x.

83. *Lyon médical,* N. 31, (Aug. 2, 1891), p 479. Henri Monod, "De l'obligation par les médecins de faire la déclaration des maladies transmissbles," *Bulletin de l'Academie de médecine,* (July 19, 1898), p 38.

84. *La France médicale et Paris médicale,* V. 39, N. 13, (Mar 25, 1893), pp 195-95; *Gazette médicale de Paris,* V. 8, N. 25, (June 10, 1891), pp 292-3.

85. A.J. Martin, *Le Concours,* V. 13, N. 38, (Sept. 19, 1891), pp 452-453.

86. G. Drouineaux, *Le Concours,* V. 1, N. 8, (August 23, 1879), pp 89-99.

87. Brouardel, *Le Secret médical,* 1887, pp 61-68.

88. *Le Concours,* V. 14, N. 31, (July 30, 1892), p 369.

89. Dr. F. de Ranse, *Gazette médicale de Paris,* V. VIII, N. 25, (June 1891), p 293; *Le Concours,* V. 9, N. 24, (June 13, 1887), p 283.

90. *Le Concours,* V. 14, N. 31, (July 30, 1892), p 369; Madame Dr. Tourangin, "Rapports avec l'Etat et les organismes dépendants de l'état." *Bul. des Soc. méd. d'Arron.,* V. 3, N. V., (Mars 5, 1900), pp 204-206.

91. R.C.C.H.P., V. 21, (1891), pp 899-901.

92. *Ibid.*

93. Brouardel, *La Profession médicale,* p 184-185.

94. J.O., 1902, pp 99-111.

95. *Gazette médicale de Paris,* V. VIII, N. 25, pp 293-94.

96. Brouardel, *La Profession médicale,* p 184.

97. Dr. H. Bourges, R.C.C.H.P., V. 30, (1900), pp 219-221. see also AN f8 170: series of communications between direction of public

assistance and public hygiene committee on how to get physicians to report cases of contagious disease, 1888-1890.

98. Brouardel, "Rapport à Monsieur le président du Conseil, Ministre de l'Intérieur," R.C.C.H.P, V. 23, (1893), pp vi-xi.

99. Brouardel, *La Professional médicale* pp 186-89.

100. Fernand Widel, "Rapport général à M. le Prés. du Conseil sur les épidémies en 1906," *Bul. de l'Academie de Médecine,* V. LIX N. 24. (June, 1908), pp 689-690.

101. Henri Monod, "Exercise de la médecine-Application de la loi du 30 Novembre 1892-Déclaration obligatoire des cas de malades épidémiques," *Rev. des Et. de Bien.,* 1894, pp 116-119.

102. "La nouvelle loi sur la protection de la santé publique," *Bul. du Syn. méd du Nord et de Pas-du-Calais* N. 1, (Jan. 1901), p 1; J. Noir, "l'Application de la loi sur la protection de la Santé publique," *Bul. Off. de l'Union des Syn. méd* N. 4, (Feb. 20, 1903), pp 57-58.

103. R.C.P.C.T., V. 2, June 1906, pp 193-194.

104. "La nouvelle loi sur la protection de la santé publique," *Bul. du syn. méd. du Nord et de Pas-de-Calais,* N. 1, (Jan, 1901), p 15; J. Noir, "l'Application de la loi sur la protection de la Santé publique," *Bul. Off. de l'Union des Syn. méd* N. 4, (Feb. 20, 1903), pp 57-58.

105. Henri Monod, "La Loi du 15 Fevrier 1902, et la déclaration des maladies transmissibles," *Revue philanthropique,* Vol 17, (1905) pp 281-297.

CHAPTER IV
THE CREATION OF A
NATIONAL MEDICAL ASSISTANCE PROGRAM*

The intent of the Medical Assistance law of July 15, 1893 was to bring licensed, official, medical care to a large sector of rural France. The law was part of the solidarist program to preserve and improve the rural population. It mandated departmental programs to pay for the medical care of indigent peasants, but the true aims of the law went beyond this. Doctors and bureaucrats believed that by providing a base clientele of indigents, the law would attract doctors to rural areas which had no resident practitioners and thus make licensed medical care available to a broader sector of the rural population. For doctors this program was a way of overcoming the perceived problem of overcrowding in the profession. The medical Assistance Law was promoted by the physicians' Union as a way of underwriting private medical care in rural areas. Although it was a government program, the Union insisted that state funds be spent in a way that maintained the private, market-orientated model of medical care. Thus, the Medical Assistance Law, in the Union's view, was a way of opposing any sort of institutional medical care, provided by hospital and dispensaries. Most importantly, the Union used the Medical Asistance Law to destroy the pre-existing cantonal systems for indigent care.

The Medical Assistance Law of 1893 was aimed primarily at rural France since by the late nineteenth century most French cities had bureaucracies and institutions which provided medical care for indigents. Most urban indigents were cared for by France's extensive urban hospital system. Many of these hospitals were connected to the Faculties of Medicine and the *Ecoles pratique de médecine*. [1] In addition to the hospitals, the urban *Bureau de bienfaisance* often provided medical assistance to indigents. However, this still left vast numbers of rural indigents with no medical aid. In 1888 15,250 communes had bureaus and 19,111 communes did not. Over half of the population lived in communes without bureaus and in many small communes the bureau existed on paper only. [2] Most bureaux which had medical assistance programs employed *médecins-fonctionnaires;* however, in Lyon and Paris the *bureau de bienfaisance* provided medical aid through home care programs that employed neighborhood general practitioners. [3] In Paris a home care system was created after considerable lobbying on the part of private physicians as a challenge to the free care provided by the Paris hospitals. [4] Opposition to free clinics was, as we have seen, common among urban private physicians who felt the hospitals took away their clients. [5] Rural doctors were no more anxious than their urban brothers to see the spread of hospital free care. Like Paris practitioners, the provincial physicians' syndicats insisted that medical assistance be based upon home care and not institutional care. Moreover, syndicat doctors wanted to have this home care provided in a way which replicated liberal, private medicine.

The development of a national medical assistance program in 1893 was in part the result of a long history of efforts by officials in some departments to provide medical care for indigents. By the late 1880s medical assistance programs existed in forty-four departments, although few of them encompassed the entire department. These programs were created in part by local initiative and in part as a result of the encouragement of the Ministry of Interior during the first decade of the Second Empire. [6] The most common form of organization was the cantonal system which originated in Alsace. [7] Under the cantonal system one or two doctors, usually called the *médecin cantonal,* were appointed by the prefect and *Conseil général* of a department to serve the indigents of a canton. The doctors were paid a yearly stipend and were obliged to treat local people who were officially enlisted as indigents by a cantonal commission. The cantonal system amounted to a pre-paid medical care program for the poor, financed by the local government. As such it was thoroughly abhorrent to the physicans' Union movement. Of the departmental medical assistance systems in place in 1887, sixty per cent had cantonal systems in operation in the entire department and another ten per cent used the cantonal system in parts of the department. [8]

Often these pre-1893 medical assistance programs were attached to other nascent public health services such as vaccination, public health council, *enfants assistés* (needy children's services) and epidemic services. The program for *enfants assistés* was the most widely organized and applied of these programs, and the only one embodied in a law *(the Loi Roussel)*. Although health reformers argued that the *Loi Roussel* was a dead letter due to lack of enforcement provisions, most departments at least appointed an inspector of the service and named doctors to posts of surveillance and monitoring. These doctor-inspectors were the only agents of national public assistance in most departments. [9] In many areas which had a program for *enfants assistés,* medical assistance was provided by the needy children's doctor *(médecin des enfants assistés)* expanding his role to include the families of the children enlisted under the program. In addition to the *médecin cantonal* and *médecin des enfants assistés,* there were a variety of other bureacratic posts such as *médecin rural, médecin de Bureau de bienfaisance, médecin des pauvres, médecin d'Assistance publique, médecin de charité, médecin du service sanitaire.* [10] *As the titles imply, in many departments these physicians were true médecins-fonctionnaires with multiple duties.*

In some cases the duties of the *médecins-fonctionnaires* were quite extensive. They were charged with broad public health responsibilities including quarantine, vaccination, handling epidemics and reporting the causes of unhealthy conditions, in addition to surveillance of *enfants assistés* and visits to public schools and the elderly. In Aisne, the *médecins de bienfaisance* were assistants to the *médecins des épidémies* and reported to the *Conseils d'hygiène* of their arrondissement on general public health concerns. In Basses-Alpes the *médecins cantonaux* were responsible for the surveillance of *enfants assistés*, visits to persons suspected of mental illness, general public health, vaccination, and admissions of ill indigents to spas. In Hautes-Alpes, the *médecins cantonaux* were responsible for vaccination, mental illness, public health and verification of cause of death. In Indre, the *Médecins du Bureau de bienfaisance* were responsible for monitoring public and private schools, manufacturing concerns and *ateliers*. In addition, they were suppose to make visits to *enfants assistés* and indigent orphans, to report on general hygiene and public health, and to report cases of epidemics and take measures to combat them. Finally, there were charged with the verification of cause of death. [11]

Some departments used rural dispensaries to provide medical care in the absence of resident doctors and pharmacists. Seine-Inférieure claimed to have created the first rural dispensary system in France. This system was modeled after successful clinics in le Havre and Rouen, two of the most progressive of French cities in public health matters. The dispensaries provided baths and showers, had regular free consultation hours, and provided limited in-patient care with emergency provisions for epidemics. They also dispensed medications and supplies, especially clean linens, for the sick. [12] In Lozére, Isére, Haute-Loire and Haute-Garonne, dispensaries were used to provide medical assistance to rural cantons that were without resident pharmacists and doctors. A visiting doctor, who was paid a fixed stipend, was available on certain days, usually two days a week. Vaccination services and emergency epidemics services were also attached to the dispensaries. [13]

In Eure-et-Loir a very extensive dispensary system was established in the 1880s by a private bequest (the Texier-Gallos foundation). There were seven dispensaries completed in 1889. They provided one or two bed in-patient care, outpatient care by visiting doctors, public baths and showers, pharmacy, surgical equipment; and had one permanent staff member. Private funds were supplemented by communal resources and the functioning of the system was overseen by a permanent commission of the *Conseil général.* In two of the cantonal dispensaries the service was hampered by the inability to find doctors who would work there, but the other five dispensaries were functioning successfully by 1895. The 1893 Medical Assistance Law, however, helped bring this system to an end. [14]

In 1889-90, in an effort to demonstrate the need for more medical assistance for the poor, the National Public Assistance Council (C.S.A.P.: Conseil supérieur de l'Assistance publique) sent out several general inspectors to survey the medical care situation in communes which did not have in any medical assistance programs. The inspectors reported on six communes whose situations they felt to be representative of the state of rural indigents and of the problem the Medical Assistance Law was to be aimed at solving. [15] The inspectors found considerable distress among rural indigents who suffered from a wide variety of chronic and acute illnesses and had no recourse to licensed practitioners. The inspectors also reported that in addition to medical problems, indigents were lacking in the basic necessities of life: adequate shelter and warmth and certainly enough food.

Commune "A" (the names of the communes were not revealed) with a population of 698 had no assistance program of any kind and no medical care available. There was no doctor in the area, not even a visiting one, and no pharmacist or religious order. Commune B of 3,303 population, the *chef-lieu* of a canton, had a *Société de sécours mutuel* (mutual insurance society) for workers who contributed one to one and a half francs a month to be cared for by a doctor who received an annual stipend of five hundred francs. This commune also had an arrangement with a nearby hospital to provide care for its indigents in cases of acute illness, but there were no provisions for chronic illness or permanent disability or non-acute illness. The inspectors reported that several elderly people in this community begged each day for bread and that two young blind children of indigent families were without medical care or education. [16]

In "Commune C", population 1,517, there was a budget of five hundred francs for general aid to a list of twenty-three indigents, nineteen of whom were widows. The local doctor, who was also a *conseiller-général,* visited these indigents free of charge. An order of nuns who resided in the community also distributed remedies among the people but the inspectors felt the nuns charged overly high prices. In spite of the commune's provisions for assisting the needy, the inspectors found several deserving families without aid. In one family the father had been without work for three months because of paralysis caused by a brain tumor. He was formerly the member of a *Société de sécours mutuel* but his aid had run out after one month. His wife was supporting their three children by doing laundry, at fifteen *sous* a day and the oldest child suffered from anemia due to malnutrition. Two other neighboring familes were in similar situations: the fathers without work due to accidents or illness, the mother doing laundry and one or more sick or aged-incapacitated family members without either medical care or adequate food. [17]

In "Commune D", population 6,175, there was no doctor in the whole canton. On Sundays the community was visited by a physician who had regular consultation hours for paying clients and would occasionally give free service to a needy person if he was without other clients. There were several illegal practitioners residing in the area and a group of nuns who ran the local girls' school and also dispensed simple home-made remedies and cared for the poor. The inspectors noted that the nuns were practicing medicine illegally, yet their medical practice was supported by a yearly stipend from the state. A bonesetter also practiced illegally in the commune. There was no licensed midwife; two "reputable matrons" regularly assisted at childbirths. The commune did occasionally send poor indigents to the departmental hospital; however, this program was poorly applied: the mayor, rather than a doctor, made the decision on who was to be sent. Thus, although modern medical care was available for paying clients, the poor of this commune, noted the inspectors, "fall in the hands of ignorance and empiricism." [18]

In "Commune F" there were 810 inhabitants, all poor mountain folk existing on about sixty francs a year and a diet of bread and potatoes. The mayor, himself a poor farmer, estimated that there were fifteen indigents in the community. When asked why there was no official list of the needy, he responded, "Why make one where there is nothing to give them. When people here are sick," he explained, "they treat themselves, usually with tisane." [19] The nearest doctor lived six kilometres away over rough ground and charged eight francs per visit. People only called him in desperate cases and then it was usually too late. Eight francs, the mayor pointed out, was the equivalent of a months food for one family in the area. When the peasants called the doctor, he added, they did not truly expect that he could help but only were reluctant to have their neighbors think that they had let a family member die without doing all they could. [20]

According to the inspectors' reports, the worst cases of indigency in these communes were among the elderly and families who had lost their principal breadwinners. These people usually lacked food and shelter as well as medical care. Elderly people were found living in hovels or in back rooms without heat or light, surviving on a diet of thin soup and bread. [21] The reports were a litany of malnourishment, blindness, epilepsy, and mental retardation. This investigation into the actual situation of France's indigents residing in communes without *bureaux de bienfaisance* or medical assistance certainly showed a clear need for medical care. However, the report indicated that starvation, malnutrition, unemployment and lack of decent housing were the most pressing problems facing these indigents. In the absence of such basic requirements for good health, the benefits of home care from a physician were questionable.

Nevertheless, in 1888 the public assistance council chose medical assistance as its top priority. Thus medical assistance became the first nationwide assistance program in France, leaving aside the rather ineffectual *Loi Roussel*. It is clear that assistance to the poor was not the only and perhaps not even the primary aim of this program. Medical assistance was intended rather to promote licensed care by doctors and to provide state support for a program which would drive out traditional practitioners such as bonesetters, nuns, and midwives. Medical assistance can be seen as a form of welfare for doctors, and therefore one could argue that the modern welfare state began with welfare programs for the bourgeoisie.

In supporting a rural medical assistance program based on private care, the C.S.A.P. of 1888 reoriented the national public welfare program in several important ways. Since the late eighteenth century national public assistance funds had been channeled primarily towards urban indigents, particularly in Paris. Since the early Third Republic some special attention was allocated to indigent children. The most striking characteristic of national assistance before 1888 was its overwhelming emphasis on institutions and bureaucratic agencies. The C.S.A.P. administered France's hospitals and asylums which took up the greatest share of its attention and monies. In addition, it provided funding and some oversight functions for the local *bureaux de bienfaisance*.

In 1885, the total budget for public assistance in France, including the state, departments and communes, was 184,121,097 francs. The assistance budget for Paris alone was 42,527,859 francs, or twenty-three per cent of the total budget, at a time when the population of Paris was about five per cent of the total French population. Assistance expenditures equaled about 2.33 francs per inhabitant in 1885; however, the funds were quite unevenly distributed between Paris and the rest of the nation: 13.54 francs per person in Paris and 1.60 francs per person in the rest of France. [22]

The state budget for assistance in 1885 emphasized hospitals, asylums and services for needy children. Institutions accounted for twenty-three per cent of the state budget; the program for *enfants assistés* and *protection des enfants du premier age* accounted for thirty-six per cent and the program for *crèches* and *sociétés de charité maternelle* accounted for another three per cent for a total of thirty-nine per cent for children's services. Eleven per cent of the budget was allocated for the *Bureau de bienfaisance* and other private institutions of a similar nature; three per cent for direct aid to indigents; and nineteen per cent for miscellaneous aid. [23]

Of the departmental budgets, forty-two per cent went toward programs to aid children and infants, and forty per cent was allocated to support permanent asylum inhabitants. Vaccination received sixteen per cent, and medical care, one per cent. [24]

The Medical Assistance Law was innovative in that it both rejected bureaucratic care and created a program which provided care for a general rural population. This meant that unlike most of their urban cousins, rural indigents would receive private medical care.

The history of the Medical Assistance Law goes back to the early Third Republic. Inspired by concern over depopulation, the first legislature of the Third Republic appointed a commission to study assistance, consisting of deputies Theophile Roussel, Lestourgie, Eugene Tallon and Morvan. [25] This commission made several legislative recommendations, including a plan for a national medical assistance program devised by Deputy Tallon. Tallon's plan called for a centralized program under the contol of the national government and based upon the existing cantonal systems. This project was not pursued and the only programs to come out of the investigation was the *Loi Roussel,* the 1873 law on public drunkenness, and the 1874 law on working children. [26]

In the 1870s, the extensive commentary on depopulation began to stress the problem of the shift of population from rural to urban areas. The principal source of populationist ideology was the *Société de la statistique de Paris,* to which many prominant Public Health Committee and national public assistance committee members belonged. [27] In several articles appearing in the society's journal between 1880 and 1884, Toussaint Loua, the statistician and populationist, delineated the problem. Loua pointed out that between 1861 and 1876 urban France had gained 618,888 inhabitants wile rural France had lost 417,308. [28] The Abbé Tounissoux of the same society indicated that this development had profound social, moral and agricultural consequences. He argued that families in rural areas were fundamentally more "...honest, decent, and religious," and further, that the migration of people to urban areas was having a disastrous effect on the morals and character of the French, particularly of French women, as placid peasants were transformed into recalcitrant workers. Tounissoux noted that Republican politicians had also taken note of the problem, even Jules Simon had said, "'La femme, devenue ouvriére, n'est plus une femme." [29] Tounissoux characterized urban society as dissolute and tending toward anarchy. [30] Contemporary observers attributed the depopulation of the countryside to the ongoing agricultural crisis of the late 1880s and early 1890s. In the hard-hit rural department of Isére, for example, the population declined by one-fourth in the 1890s. [31] This anxiety over the decline of the rural population was part of the general concern over the political and social consequences of an expanding urban working class. [32]

State bureaucrats and departmental officials argued that rural people were attracted to the cities in part because of the greater availability of medical and social assistance there. [33] For example, the C.S.A.P. reported that the *Conseils généraux* of Aisne and Haute-Marne, two departments which had lost population to more urban departments, attributed their losses to the absence of social services in the countryside. According to M. Mongeot of the *Conseil général* of Haute- Marne, the emigrants moved to the city to find medical and social aid, but instead of finding better health, "...the robust and healthy [rural] population arrives to sicken and die in the atmosphere of the city." [34] Brouardel noted that the abolition of the *officiers de santé* worsened the medical care situation in the countryside and made medical assistance programs all the more necessary to attract doctors to replace the current *officiers* as they died. [35]

In 1888 medical assistance became a major topic of discussion among the government and public assistance bureaucracy. The C.S.A.P. began to draft a law and to make recommendations for the implementation of medical assistance programs. Thus medical assistance joined medical practice and public health as major legislative issues of the late 1880s and early 1890s. All three of these issues should be interpreted as part of a general solidarist program to unify the nation and to placate social unrest by giving the lower classes a reason to support the still shaky Third Republic. Public assistance bureaucrats and national legislators justified medical assistance on humanitarian, nationalist-populationist, and historic grounds, noting that the constituent assembly of the Revolution had declared that assistance was "...a primary duty...commanded by the natural rights of a society." Henri Monod and Minister of the Interior Floquet called up historical precedent for state assistance. They reminded the government that Henry II had begun the important task of taking assistance away from the church by expanding the role of the state, and that the revolutionary assembly of 1790 had intended to expand assistance programs to reach all French people. [36] The plans of the *Comité pour l'extinction de la mendacité* of 1790, however, had envisioned a national program of basic welfare assistance for indigents, a plan which was later revived during the short-lived Second Republic. [37] The solidarist program of the Third Republic was quite different from these earlier ideas concerning social assistance. The solidarists concentrated on specific rather than comprehensive programs, aiming first at needy children and public drunkenness, and then at medical care. The law on medical assistance was a step beyond the *Loi Roussel* in that it was made legally binding on the departments which were required to create budgets for the medical assistance program. The *Loi Roussel* was optional, but the Medical Assistance Law was not. Moreover, medical assistance had the backing of an increasingly powerful public assistance bureaucracy, as well as the local physicians' syndicats equally determined to see the law put into effect. The result was that medical assistance was the first really effective national public assistance program. It is interesting that this social program provided professional medical care, the effectiveness of which was questionable to say the least, but ignored the basic necessities of life which so many of the poor clearly lacked. The program was made possible because Solidarists argued that this unprecedented government intervention into formerly private concerns was justified on the grounds that the general interests of the nation overruled any other considerations.

Henri Monod, director of public assistance in 1888, argued that assistance had to be legally enacted in order to force the compliance of local governments which up to that point had largely abandoned their sick indigents. Monod argued that medical assistance would benefit the nation economically by preserving the population. "To increase the chances for recovery of a sick person who lives from his labor is to contribute to safeguarding the most precious capital of a country, that of its lives."[38] Emile Rey who presented the law to the legislature observed that

"Medical assistance for the poor is the workshop for the repair of the most important machinery of national work, human machinery. We must remember that contrary to what is going on among our enemies, it seems that this equipment renews itself more and more slowly, it seems as if we are menaced by diminishing growth; who can help but feel patriotic anguish when he learns that the excess of births over deaths, which has been declining for a number of years, last year reached a deficit? National defense itself risks being profoundly hampered and the world influence of France seriously compromised."[39]

The Public Assistance Council drew an analogy between medical assistance and the recent law on universal primary education. "To assure benefits to the whole population it is necessary to make it a legal obligation. If this principle is acceptable in public education it is also acceptable in medical assistance."[40]

In his report in the name of the special subcommittee on medical assistance, Dr. Dreyfus-Brisac referred to the arguments of Theophile Roussel and La Rochefoucauld-Liancourt, head of the *Comité pour l'extinction de la mendacité* of 1790, both of whom pointed out the benefits to the state of promoting assistance programs. La Rochefoucauld-Liancourt said the state had a responsibility to aid ill workers and children "in moral danger," because they were the future workers of society and, further, that the state should aid indigent elderly and permanently incapacitated workers because they had provided a life of labor for the nation. [41] In the legislative discussions on the Medical Assistance Law, this notion of a right to assistance was an important argument in favor of the bill. [42] The idea of duty was reciprocal, however, for the duty of society to care for its workers was balanced by the workers' duty to labor for the nation.

The C.S.A.P. emphasized the concept of reciprocal duty over right, a distinction Roussel made in his arguments for the 1872 law to protect infants. [43] In other words, the poor did not have the right to expect assistance unless they fulfilled their duty to work. However this duty did not, in the minds of the Public Assistance Council, justify programs of forced work such as existed in the provisions of the British and German public welfare programs. While the French Public Assistance Council admired the effectiveness of the Poor Law of Britain in keeping the number of indigents on public assistance down, they were opposed to forced labor in principle. They pointed out that the British system, in spite of many modifications, was expensive to maintain and abhorrent from the standpoint of personal liberty. A note of national conceit entered these observations as Dreyfus-Brisac noted that ideas of social solidarity and general social humanitarianism had not made an impact in Britain as they had in France. [44]

The Medical Assistance Law of 1893 was the first major project of the C.S.A.P. (Conseil supérieur de l'Assistance publique), created in April 1888 under the Ministry of the Interior. The C.S.A.P.'s first director was Henri Monod. A year later the Public Health Committee was transferred from the Ministry of Agriculture and Commerce to the

Ministry of Interior and also placed under Monod's direction. [45]

Monod was formerly prefect of Finistére where he took special interest in the health and public assistance problems of that department. In 1892 he published a work on cholera in Finistére. [46] Monod, along with Bourardel, occupied a position of great influence in the government in medical and public assistance matters. Although the private physicians' syndicats were sometimes in conflict with him over issues such as the abolition of the *officiers de santé*, (which he subsequently ceased opposing) and the declaration of epidemic diseases, Monod was lauded by Auguste Cézilly in 1891 for his support of the medical profession. Monod was also a vice president of the *société de protection des victimes du devoir médical*, an organization created by Le Concours to give aid to families of doctors who died as a result of their practice. [47] During the formulation, enactment, and implementation of the law, Monod kept in close touch with the leaders of the Union of Syndicats and of Le Concours. [48]

Doctors made up a large portion of the membership of the C.S.A.P. The subcommittee of this body which drew up the plans for the Medical Assistance Law had eighteen members, fifteen of whom were doctors. [49] Two of the members who were very active in formulating the plans for medical assistance were Dr. Gibert, Mayor of Le Havre, and Dr. Lardier of the Vosges. Gibert was also very active in the society *Le Concours médical*. He received a special thanks at the October 1889 general assembly of that society for his services. He was a past president of the le Havre medical syndicat and honorary president of the

Union. [50] Lardier was also an active member of Le Concours who received special recognition at the 1889 general assembly and was the long-time president of the medical syndicat of the Vosges. [51]

At its first general assembly in January 1887 the Union decided to made medical assistance legislation a top priority. Spokesmen at the assembly declared their intention to reorganize the cantonal medical assistance systems which already existed in about 50% of the nation's departments. Syndicat doctors complained that cantonal assistance was dominated by the elites of the profession, especially "those with scientific titles," who excluded the ordinary doctor from government programs. [52] The Union doctors also claimed that cantonal medical programs, like other bureaucratic health position, were an electoral gold mine for "physician-politicians who often have turned to politics because they are incapable of competing successfully with their brothers on the basis of medical skills." [53] For the private doctor it was crucial that medical assistance be kept separate from pre-existing state medical programs such as vaccination, inspection of schools and services for needy children. Further, the private doctors argued that medical assistance should be kept separate from the still rudimentary but growing public health programs. [54] Rather than see it remain a mainstay of bureaucratic medicine, the Union believed they could re-structure medical assistance so that it supported liberal, private, professional medicine. In order to do so, medical assistance would have to protect and promote what practitioners in the Union movement called the independence and freedom of doctors and patients. For private practitioners this meant that doctors would be free to choose to participate or not in medical assistance programs. They argued as well that patients cared for under the system should have a choice of doctors. Union doctors pointed out their goals were in direct opposition to the continued existence of the "médecin-fonctionnaires," created by the hospital system, the *Loi Roussel,* and cantonal medical assistance programs.

In addition to being a way of destroying cantonal medicine, the Union saw medical assistance in revised form as a way of advancing the terrain of the private practitioner into areas which had previously been too poor, or perhaps simply unwilling, to support licensed medicine. [55] To achieve both these ends it was crucial to the Union that medical assistance not be centralized under the state bureaucracy. They feared that such centralization would increase the power of the elite Parisian physicians of the Faculty of Medicine and the Academy of Medicine who heretofore had been the dominant influence on the government in medical planning and who had furthermore helped create the *médecins-fonctionnaires.* [56]

Medical assistance was a major topic at all the annual meetings of the society *Le Concours* and the *Union des syndicats* between 1888-1893. In 1890 Dr. Lassalle justified the doctors' lobbying efforts in favor of their version of the bill in language which reflects the general attitude of the syndicat doctors toward medical legislation at this time:

> "...until now, we [the private doctors] have always been considered to be obligated and responsible to perform charity and that has been our fault. We see the other professions obtain

concessions and advantages because they have cried out a great deal. I maintain that if we, private doctors, would agitate as they do, given the influence which we possess with our deputies and those for whom we have often been the major electoral agents, we would obtain the enactment of our modest and just demands." [57]

As soon as the C.S.A.P. took up the question of medical assistance, it asked the Union to form an advisory commission. In February of 1888, the Union appointed Drs. Gassot, Leroy, Lardier, Maurat, Millet, Margueritte, Dupuy and Mignen to this commission. The commission argued that all communes should be legally required to have medical assistance programs but that the organization should be left up to each department to determine. The commission emphasized that the freedom of doctor and patient should be maintained, the former to choose to participate or not, the latter to choose which practitioner he would visit. Further, they stated that the practitioner should be paid according to the amount of services rendered, specifically that he should be paid a fee for each visit to a patient. They argued that the function of assistance physician should be kept separate from pre-existing medical and welfare services such as vaccination, school inspection, epidemic services. They stated that doctors of each commune or department should have the responsibility of organizing the service in their area. Finally, the commission argued that medical assistance should be a home care program which would put restraints on the establishment of cantonal hospitals and reserve hospital care for "exceptional" cases. [58]

The syndicat commission also sought to limit the number of people eligible for treatment under the system by prohibiting families paying six francs a year in taxes from participating. The commission also recommended that the C.S.A.P. subcommittee look at Loiret and the Vosges for the best examples of how medical assistance should function. [59]

With his positions on both the Union commission and on the subcommittee of the C.S.A.P. responsible for writing the law, Dr. Lardier was an important connection between the interests of the syndicat doctors and the creators of the medical assistance legislation. He characterized his function on the subcommittee to the readers of *Le Concours* as

"...the defender of medical liberty and the independence which can be enhanced or diminished by various parts of the proposed law. I must add that thanks to the syndicats who are becoming more and more united and vigorous, I believe that the rights of doctors will be adequately protected." [60]

At the request of his colleagues at *Le Concours,* Lardier submitted an amendment to the subcommittee which he hoped would further protect the liberty of doctors under the medical assistance program. It stated that once a doctor had participated in his departments medical assistance program, he could not be eliminated from the program unless gross misconduct was proven. Lardier explained, "The absolute independence of the doctor must be protected if society expects to call on his devotion and sacrifice." [61] The subcommittee disapproved his amendment, however, because it interfered too much with the local control over medical assistance.

Lardier attempted, also unsuccessfully, to get another *Le Concours* project accepted by the C.S.A.P. subcommittee. This amendment would have required all doctors in a given commune, or association of communes constituting a medical assistance circumscription, to be on the commissions which drew up the lists of indigents. Gassot defend this stipulation on the grounds that "the doctor, better than anyone else, knows the true poor because he goes daily to their homes and knows the character of the people, those who flaunt and those who hide their poverty." [62] This idea was again rejected by the C.S.A.P. subcommittee, but came up again when the law was discussed in the Senate in March 1893. Senator-Dr. Andre Victor Cornil obliged *Le Concours* and the Union by again proposing the Lardier-Gassot amendment, this time to the Senate. Several Senators objected that it amounted to a conflict of interest to have physicians participate so closely in the administration of a bill which directly affected their personal welfare. Gassot argued that these objections were ridiculous and insisted that doctors would only act in the interest of the smooth functioning of the service. [63] Cornil withdrew the amendment when at the request of Cézilly and Dr. Porsons, the Vice-President of the *Union des syndicats,* Monod agreed that in practice the C.S.A.P. would see to it that doctors be consulted in the making of the lists of eligible indigents. [64]

The Union commission was very concerned that the role of dispensaries in medical assistance be kept minimal. Gassot was outraged that dispensaries were mentioned at all in the text of the law. According to Gassot, the law suggested that communes could build dispensaries where doctors would be available for consultations to indigents. Gassot objected to this strongly as too heavy a burden on doctors. Instead he favored the idea that doctors give consultations in their homes or make visits to the patient's home, which meant that the doctor would decide when and under what circumstance he would examine his indigent patient. [65] Lardier reassured Gassot that the proposed text of the law only required comunes to make arrangements with the nearest hospital or dispensary for the care of their poor in those cases where they could not adequately be cared for by the local doctor in their own homes. The indigents would be admitted to the hospital only with the permission of their doctor. Lardier emphasized that such cases would be "exceptional." [66]

For the Union the most important function of the new Medical Assistance Law was the elimination of the cantonal system of medicine. The syndicats indentified cantonal doctors as the incarnation of all the evils of state medicine; they were the worst example of the *médecin-fonctionnaire.* [67] Private doctors also believed that the cantonal system robbed them of clients by treating people who were not truly indigent. [68] Physicians in the Union felt that by their mere existence cantonal doctors threatened the profession by practicing in a way which was contrary to the principles of private practice. According to Union ideology there was no room in the profession for doctors who did not conform to private practice. The cantonal doctors were of course paid by stipend and thus were under obligations to the state who paid them and to the people for whom they were charged to care. As the Union saw it, such doctors lost the liberty to choose whether to give or with-hold treatment, a privilege to which the private doctors clung tena-ciously.

Paul Brouardel agreed with the Union that cantonal medicine was dangerous to the profession. As far back as 1873 Brouardel had claimed that the cantonal system "...takes away our liberty...Peasants never learn that medicine is a free profession." [69] Long-standing oppo-sition to cantonal medicine also existed among the private practitioners of Paris where free home care existed in most arrondissements. Paris physicians had organized successfully to pressure the municipal council to keep the position of the *Médecins du Bureau de bienfaisance* open to any doctors who wished to participate. [70]

In 1887 the leaders the Union and *Le Concours* launched a feverish campaign to lobby for their version of medical assistance with the C.S.A.P., the government and departmental authorities. Their major task was to create the sort of medical assistance programs they supported, and arguments in support of them, before the law was enacted. Then they would be able to present these programs and as models to harried prefects and *Conseils généraux* when these local officials were con-fronted with the legal requirement to implement medical assistance. [71] The model which the Union adopted was known as the Landais system after the department of Landes where it was evidently first organized. Created in 1856 by a committee of local doctors in Landes, this system replicated private practice in several crucial ways. All practitioners in a given area were allowed to participate if they so chose, indigents were given a choice of practitioner, and most importantly, the practitioners were paid by the visit. It is unclear how long the Landais system ever functioned in the department of its birth, for by 1885, according to a report to the C.S.A.P., the system was no longer working according to the way it had been originally developed. According to the report, doctors in the department of Landes were not free to choose to participate in the system but rather were appointed by the prefect. Furthermore, only a portion of the departmental communes still paid them by the visit. [72] The promoters of the Landais system did not publicize this fact; rather they continually cited the Landais system as originally developed as the model form of medical assistance for national adoption.

Le Concours and the Union urged fellow syndicalists to take up the argument of the Union against the *médecins-fonctionnaries* and cantonal system and to use the influence of their local medical press and syndicats on their departmental governments in favor of the Landais system. [73] Dr. Grellety even composed a poem on the subject entitled, "Les intérêts des médecins et le project de loi sur l'assistance publique dans les départements," [74] In 1888-89 doctors belonging to *Le Concours* and the Union set up Landais type medical assistance systems in Loiret, Oise, Seine-et-Oise, Loire-Inférieure and Vienne. In anticipation of the law on medical assistance, Union doctors publicized these programs as better alternatives to cantonal medicine. In fact, like the original system in Landes, these departmental systems functioned very poorly or not at all.

Dr. Porson, president of the *Syndicat médical de la Loire-Inférieure* created a Landais system for his department and wrote several articles in *Le Concours* between 1888-93 praising its virtues. However, the system was not put into effect until 1895. [75] Dr. Gassot of Loiret criticized Porson's system which he claimed involved too much paper work and too much mayoral involvement. Gassot advocated a modified version of the Landais system which he had recently put into effect in Loiret, replacing a cantonal system which had been established in 1852. Under Gassot's system, medical assistance doctors were selected by all the private doctors in a given area and were paid a fee based upon the number of indigents in their charge and upon the distance traveled to treat them. Gassot argued that this preserved the dignity of doctors and preserved their independence from clients and from local officials, mayors in particular. [76] Gassot's refinement of the Landais system was not popular among the leaders of *Le Concours* and Union because it was too close to the old cantonal system. [77]

Like Porsons, Doctors Fourmestreaux and Maurat of the Seine-et-Oise syndicat created a Landais system in their department which they publicized as models of medical assistance. Although Fourmestreaux and Maurat described their Landais systems in glowing terms, their systems never ran smoothly and were, on the contrary, the cause of much strife between the syndicat doctors and departmental and local officials. [78] By 1899, the Landais system was no longer opperating in the department, and a substantial portion of the communes had reverted to cantonal practices of yearly stipends as their method of paying doctors. [79] Dr. Mignen, also of the Union and president of the doctors' syndicat of Montaigue (Vendée), publicized the Landais system he created in the Vendée in the late 1880s. [80] By 1895, however, this system was in considerable difficulty as doctors' bills greatly exceeded the department's budget and the administration began making proportional reductions in payments to doctors. [81] The Landais program in Vienne, also established in 1888, suffered from similar problems. [82]

In Cézilly's home department, Oise, the Landais program also ran into great difficulties. Although enacted at the departmental level, it was rejected by a majority of the communes, which retained the cantonal system. By 1895 the system was still not actually functioning in several arrondissements and the *Conseil général* of the department voted to end payment by visit in favor of yearly stipends, in effect re-establishing the cantonal system. [83]

Of these much publicized model Landais systems, then, only Gassot's program in Loiret, which was more like the cantonal system, was functioning successfully in 1888-95. The arguments used by *Le Concours* and the Union to promote the Landais system were based on departments where its success was highly questionable. Nevertheless the C.S.A.P. adopted the doctors' views virtually without exception and cited the same examples to support the Landais system and criticize the cantonal system. The C.S.A.P. promoted this view in spite of the fact that its own survey revealed the serious problems the Landais systems had encountered. [84]

In contrast to Tallon's proposed legislation of the early 1870s, the C.S.A.P. plan called for a decentralized system. Monod complained about the disinterest of local authorities in medical assistance, but nevertheless argued that once medical assistance was made obligatory on local authorities it should be left up to them to organize and implement. Monod also argued that decentralization would preserve local customs and make the systems more financially efficient because the same authority that was allocating funds would be spending them. [85] In supporting decentralization, members of the C.S.A.P. defined the commune as the basic unit of governmental aid for the indigent. According to their ideology, the first level of recourse for the individual was the family. In the absence of the family the duty fell to the commune. "For what is a commune, if not a large family...if the family is the first level of society, the commune is the second." [86] The only problem with making the commune responsible was the increasing mobility of French society. It became necessary for the C.S.A.P. to enact a complex series of regulations defining residency. The commune would only be responsible for the care of indigents who had lived among them at least two years. The care of indigents with no legal commune of residence under the law would fall to the responsibility of the department of residence or the state if they had been traveling among the departments. [87]

In their written text of the law, the C.S.A.P. left great latitutde to local authorities in determining the form the systems would take. However, in all the C.S.A.P.'s public comments on medical assistance, including its recommendations for systems, arguments to the legislature and directives to the departmental administrators, it only discussed home care by physicians. [88] In addition, everywhere at the local level doctors echoed this point of view so that only a few departments thought to try out dispensary or small hospital systems as a way of implementing medical assistance. In effect the law led to the demise of dispensary systems; doctors forced the adoption of Landais systems and took home care functions away from the dispensaries. [89]

According to the C.S.A.P.'s original plan, *bureaux de bienfaisance* would be created in every commune and would be responsible to draw up lists of eligible indigents. Upon further investigation into the history of the *bureaux*, the council realized this idea was impractical in a nation composed of thousands of communes some of which were made up of tiny scattered hamlets of three to four families. Thus it was ultimately left up to mayors and municipal officials to draw up lists of indigents and oversee medical assistance. This meant the further decentralization of medical assistance since the *bureaux de bienfaisance* would have had direct recourse to the prefect in case of disagreements with the local officials. [90]

How to create the lists of indigents was a critical issue, for the council recognized that all their plans could flounder due to the widespread fear in France of creating "vast armies of the poor." [91] The council estimated from the records of the functioning *bureaux de bienfaisance* that about 6.24 per cent of the French population was indigent. The council was disturbed to note that France had a much greater percentage of its population falling into the category of indigency that either Germany or Great Britain. [92] According to the C.S.A.P. report, Germany reported 2.8 per cent indigency and Britain 3.38 per cent of the population enrolled as indigent. Monod and Dreyfus-Brisac argued that Britain and Germany under-estimated their poverty and that in fact the French population was not less well off materially than either the German or British. [93] In looking at the number of indigents aided in the various departments with medical assistance programs, the council found large divergences which it claimed had little to do with the relative wealth of the departments. For example, the rate was 1.68 per cent in Doubs, 1.79 in Allier, 3.4 in Cher, 3.25 in Gers and 14.84 in Pas-de-Calais, 10.21 in the Somme and 13.6 in the Vosges. The committee decided to set a 6.45 per cent as a guideline for all departments in enlisting indigents. [94]

Dreyfus-Brisac, the chairman of the C.S.A.P. subcommittee on medical assistance, claimed that there was unanimity of opinion among the members of the subcommittee that home care was the most effective way of implementing medical assistance. He admitted, however, that there was a vast difference of opinion among the committee members over the form that home care assistance programs should take. Nonetheless his report, in the name of the whole comittee, was highly critical of the cantonal system. Dreyfus-Brisac noted that the cantonal system had been the form of medical assistance advocated by the Academy of Medicine in 1833 but since that time had been severely criticized by private physicians. He pointed out that the medical syndicats, at the time of his report, were unified in their opposition to cantonal medicine. He further claimed that even in the Haut-Rhin, the heart of the cantonal system, the *Conseil général* had recently supported the motion of a *docteur-conseiller* to revise their cantonal system. [95] In criticizing the cantonal system, Dreyfus-Brisac echoed the doctors' complaints that it created *médecins-fonctionnaires* who were far too dependant upon prefects, mayors, and the sick for their livelihood. [96] Dreyfus-Brisac also brought up the issue that cantonal system was an attack on freedom of choice in medical care. [97]

In acclaiming the Landais system, Dreyfus-Brisac illustrated the close influence which the Union movement exercised in the C.S.A.P. He repeated all the major points of the Union's position and completely ignored the C.S.A.P.'s own report on the functioning of medical assistance in the departments. Following the recommendations of the *Le Concours* committee, Dreyfus-Brisac cited the Landais systems in the Vosges and Loiret as the best examples to commend the system. However, the C.S.A.P.'s own records showed that the Vosges system was not really functioning and that the Loiret system was more like a cantonal system than a Landais. [98] Apparently forgetting his previous criticism of *médecins-fonctionnaires,* Dreyfus-Brisac pointed out that another virtue of the Landais system in the Vosges was that the participating doctors also functioned as inspectors of schools, epidemics and needy children. He concluded that the virtue of the Landais system was that it "...safeguarded the independence of the doctor, because all the doctors in any area were free to choose to take part and because the doctors were paid according to the services they rendered." [99] He also argued that the Landais system was actually more economical to operate than the cantonal system. He finally pointed out, almost as an afterthought, that the patients benefited from being able to choose their own doctor. [100]

It is questionable of course whether a choice of doctors was really available to rural indigents, since few rural communities had access to more than one doctor. [101] Local observers also doubted that rural people were really concerned about this issue and pointed out that under most of the medical assistance programs operating out of the urban *bureaux de bienfaisance,* indigents had no such right. [102]

The advocacy of home care over hospital care marked an abrupt departure from the traditional role of the assistance bureaucracy whose primary duty it had been from the late 18th century to the late 19th to oversee France's hospital system. Dreyfus-Brisac admitted that for the rural poor access to the hospital was even more difficult than access to home care by physicians. He cited the failure of the law of August 7, 1851 which had invited all communes and departments to organize hospital care for their indigents. Under that law, prefects were to divide their departments into districts based on available hospitals and set daily rates for the care of the poor. Communes were to make direct arrangements with the hospitals to pay for the care of their sick indigents. The law had no legal enforcement procedures attached and so remained a dead letter except in those departments and communes with strong interests in medical care for the poor, and these were few. Even where programs existed, communes voted inadequate funds so that ill people were not cared for long enough to truly recover. A report from the *Conseil général* of Aisne indicated that people were routinely sent home before they were able to return to work, and with no means of support they simply worsened and died. In the commune of Fossy in 1889, a peasant in this situation had committed suicide when expelled from the departmental hospital after his commune stopped paying his bills. [103] In Yonne it was said that rural communes often took their ill indigents to the cities and abandoned them on the sidewalks in front of the hospitals. [104] A study in Maine-et-Loire in 1887 reported that of 381 communes 38 possessed some sort of hospital, 102 others had arrangements to use one or two beds at a neighboring hospital and 241 communes were completely without access to hospital care. [105] Because of the communes' increasing unwillingness to pay, from 1851 on more and more urban hospitals began to refuse to care for indigents from outside their communes. [106]

In defense of the C.S.A.P. decision not to remedy the problems left by the 1851 hospital law, Dreyfus-Brisac argued that hospital care was not a viable way of providing adequate medical assistance for the countryside because of the attitudes of the rural poor. He pointed out that one of the traditions bequeathed from the Ancien Regime and enshrined by the attitudes of the social reformers of the revolutionary period was fear of hospitals. [107] This fear originated from the infamous *hôpitaux généraux* which were mainly institutions of political repression rather than medical care. Dreyfus-Brisac argued that this attitude would continue to make it difficult to establish an effective hospital system in France. [108] Henry Monod also declined to support hospitals or dispensaries as alternative means of providing rural medical assistance. [109]

A variety of evidence supports Dreyfus-Brisac's contention that hospitals continued to suffer from a bad reputation. [110] Joigneaux pointed out that villagers feared going to the hospital because of reluctance to be separated from their families and because of a fear they would die and be buried in a strange city cemetery far from the village churchyard. [111] A hospital commission in Côte-d'Or reported in 1893 that they could not be sure that if a new hospital system were built it would be used. They were considering the construction of several small hospitals in some rural cantons in the arrondissements of Dijon and Chatellain which were without access to any medical care. The commission reported that while hospitals were well accepted in the cities they were distrusted by country folk who considered the hospital only a place to die. The commission observed that this became a self-fulfilling prophecy since rural French women and men only went to hospitals as a desperate last resort. The conclusion of this commission was to build a system of dispensaries rather than hospitals. [112] In Hautes-Alpes a hospital/hospice was built in 1875 from a private bequest to serve the cantons of Tallard and Barcellonnette which had previously been without hospitals. This hospital was scarcely ever used and in 1889, the Conseil général voted to turn it into a school. [113]

Dr. Saloman of Savigne-l'Evêque in Sarthe complained that modern ideas about medical care were not in line with the attitudes of the rural poor. He said that although "modern palaces" had replaced the hospitals of the Ancien Regime, the poor patient, even when seriously ill, preferred to stay at home without care than be taken to the hospital. [114] A *conseiller-général* of Aisne reported that a commune in his area had voted a special tax to support care for a sick indigent resident at the hospital in Monteuil only to find that the indigent threatened to kill himself if he was sent there because, he stated, it amounted to being "...interned as a vagabond." [115]

The Ministry of Interior had attempted several times to survey the availability of hospital beds in France. There were enormous difficulties in arriving at an accurate picture because of the lack of interest in and knowledge of hospitals displayed by prefects and mayors. An inquiry of 1878 headed by de Crisenoy found that of 59,997 hospital beds available in rural France, 24,562 were vacant. In Calvados, 511 of 600 beds were vacant; in Meuse 400 of 619 and in Nord, 856 of 1438. An 1886 inquiry found that in rural France about twenty-two per cent of all hospice beds (10,723 of 47,964) and forty per cent of all hospital beds (15,709 of 39,248) were vacant. A study of 1889 found that of about 120,000 hospital beds in all of France outside of Paris, 35,000 were empty. [116] Dr. Elie Peyron of the C.S.A.P. subcommittee on medical assistance, observed that the under-utilization of hospital beds was not due to lack of applicants but rather resulted from the refusal of hospital commissions to admit patients from outside their communes in spite of the fact that the law of 1851 had required them to do so. [117]

There were many reasons why hospitals should have been a part of the medical assistance program. As the commission recognized, hospitals constituted a readily available resource for medical care which was not being fully utilized. It was also becoming clear at the time that the plans for medical assistance were being formulated that asepsis was making hospitals much safer. Moreover, it was easier to assure a germ-free environment in hospitals than in many homes of the lower classes. [118] Furthermore, sick indigents at home continued to be not only subject to unsanitary environment but also to cold, damp, and malnutrition. It was only in the hospitals that rural indigents could be assured of a clean bed, some heat, and adequate nutrition. In 1888 the department of Haute-Savoie had rejected home-care medical assistance and instead launched a program to build more hospitals. The departmental authorities despaired of finding enough rural doctors to care for indigents, and further argued that only in institutions could they provide adequate food and comfort. [119] Hospitals could also maintain the kind of isolation which public health authorities had realized would stop the spread of contagious disease. The public health and public assistance authorities recognized the importance of hospital care for contagious diseases, surgery, and overall adequate care, but Dreyfus-Brisac's committee completely ignored the possibility of encouraging the increased the utilization of the nation's empty hospital beds. Instead, the committee pushed ahead on its plan to create medical assistance under home care by private practitioners.

The C.S.A.P. not only pushed for home care as opposed to institutional care, but it also sponsored a type of home care program, the Landais system, whose functioning was already questionable. The council's own statistics on the functioning of medical assistance in 1887 indicated that the cantonal system served far more of the poor, at less expense, than did the Landais system. It should be pointed out, however, that the effect of medical assistance on rural indigents was never the central concern of those planning the law. Instead both doctors and public assistance authorities focused on doctors and administration. Peyron himself noted in the subcommittee discussions that the primary goal was to attract doctors to areas without licensed practitioners. [120] Indigents were discussed only in reference to setting guidelines on the numbers that should be treated.

An analysis of the statistics available for thirty-three of the forty-four departments which had medical assistance programs in 1887 indicates that for all systems the average percentage of indigents enrolled was 5.9 per cent of the participating population. For the cantonal system, however, this figure was 6.0 per cent and for the Landais, 3.0 per cent, a statistically significant difference (see Table IV-I). [121] The average enrollment of indigents under the cantonal system was also closer to the figure which the Public Assistance Council saw as the true average percentage of France's population actually in need of assistance (6.4 per cent). There was also a difference between the two systems for the percentage of indigents actually treated (measured as a percentage of the indigents enrolled), although the difference was not found to be statistically significant. Under the Landais system 26.1 per cent of those enlisted were treated, the corresponding figure for the cantonal system was 33.4 per cent (see Table IV-1). [122] This would seem a logical result of the degree of power which doctors versus indigents had over whether or not they were treated. The percentage of indigents treated under the cantonal system, 33.4, is not as out of line as it might seem since it was frequently observed that in practice communes only enlisted indigents who were actually elderly, infirm or currently ill. As the Assistance Committees survey indicated, French indigents were typically undernourished and in poor health. Further, subsequent statistics on the functioning of medical assistance in 1897-99 show that thirty-five per cent was the overall average of indigents treated from the list of indigents enrolled. [123] As far as costs are concerned, although Dreyfus-Brisac argued that cantonal care was more expensive than the Landais system, expenses for the existing Landais systems, measured as a ratio of expenses to indigents treated, were over twice that of the cantonal systems: 18.2 francs versus 8.8 francs; again, a statistically significant difference (see Table IV-1). [124]

The institution of National Medical Assistance in 1893 must be seen as welfare for the medical profession rather than welfare for the poor. In a sense, the program was a step out of its time, for the Public Assistance Council's own surveys showed that France's poor were in desperate need of food and shelter as well as in poor health. In face of such deprivation, of what worth was medical care? Further, in this era before antibiotics and sulfa drugs, and when asepsis was just beginning to penetrate into regular medical practice and germ theory was not yet widely accepted, the effectiveness of medical care by private practitioners was highly questionable.

The doctors' version of medical assistance called for departmental systems which emphasized home care over dispensaries and hospitals, in which payment would be for services rendered, and in which doctors would be able to freely choose to participate and compete for clients. In embracing and promoting this program, the Public Assistance Council was in effect creating state support for liberal, professional medicine. In doing so they made a departure from the medical assistance programs planned during the revolution, Second Republic and early Third Republic, and by endorsing decentralization adopted a system not advocated by the National Public Health Committee (C.C.H.P.). In promoting the Landais system, *Le Concours,* the Union, and finally the Public Assistance Council were advocating a system which had proven less effective in reaching the truly poor of France, and far more costly to operate than the cantonal system, an easily available and well established alternative. Nevertheless, the combination of the C.S.A.P. support with the well-organized promotions of the Union at the national and the syndicats at local level, resulted in the Landais system's becoming widely applied after medical assistance was enacted into law in 1893. The following chapter will take up the story of the consequences of medical assistance and the Landais system at the local level.

Table IV-I

Functioning of Medical Assistance Under
Different Systems in 1887
(Before the Enactment of the Medical Assistance Law)*

System	Number of Departments	Indigents Eligible: Average Percent of Total Population	Indigents Treated: Average Percent of Indigents Eligible	Average Expenses per Indigent Treated
Landais	4	3.0%	26.1%	18.17 francs
Cantonal	22	6.0%	33.4%	8.80 francs
Mixed	7	4.2%	42.2%	18.89 francs
All	33	5.3%	34.4%	12.07 francs

*Conseil superieur d'Assistance publique, Fascicule 9, Tableaux I,II. Archives de la Sante publique, Paris. Two departments in this report were left out of the statistical study: Corse, because its medical assistance system was organized along Italian traditions, and Vosges, because its system was not functioning according to the report itself.

Note: The Mann-Whitney test of central tendency was used, due to small sample size, to test the significance of the differences between the means for the Landais and Cantonal systems. Significance was accepted at the <.05 level. The difference in the means between the Landais and Cantonal systems for Indigents Eligible and for Expenses per Indigent Treated was found to be significant. The difference in the means for Indigents Treated was not found to be statistically significant. Calculations were done on a Prime computer using the Statistical Package for the Social Sciences.

NOTES TO CHAPTER IV

*The tables and some of the material in this and the following chapter appear in my article: "Medical Rivalries and Medical Politics in France: The Physicians' Union Movement and the Medical Assistance Law of 1893," Forthcoming: *Journal of the History of Medicine and Allied Sciences,* January, 1987.

1. Michel Foucault, *The Birth of the Clinic* 1972; Erwin Ackernecht, *Medicine at the Paris Hospital,* 1967.

2. Henri Monod, "Assistance médicale dans les Campagnes," *Conseil supérieur de l'Assistance publique, Fasiscule 22,* p 10; (hereinafter C.S.A.P., Fasc. 22). According to the *Gazette médicale de Paris,* the number of communes prossessing bureaux de bienfaisance was 14,871, *Gazette médicale de Paris,* S.7, V.Vi, N.42, (Oct. 9, 1889), p 503. The history of the *Bureaux de bienfaisance* goes back to the *Bureaux de charité* of the Ancien Régime. The *Bureaux de charité* were created by proclamations issued by Henry II in 1536 and 1544 which also insti-tuted a poor tax and created a *Bureau central des pauvres.* In 1790, under the leadership of La Rochefoucauld-Liancort of the *Comité pour l'extinction de la mendacité,* the Revolutionary Assembly planned to

create a national assistance network which would reach all French men and women. However these plans were scaled down under the Directory. The law of 7 Frimaire, An 5, required only municipalities of over 2000 in population to have *Bureaux de bienfaisance:*. C.S.A.P. Fasc. 22; M. Floquet, Minister of Interior, "Discours-Séance d'Inauguration, Conseil supérieur de l'Assistance publique," *Le Concours médical,* (hereinafter Le Concours) V. 10, N. 25, (June 23, 1888) pp 294-99.

3. Jeanne Gaillard, "Assistance et urbanisme dans les Paris de Second Empire" *Récherches* (Fontenay sous-bois) N. 29 (1977) p 395.

4. "l'Assistance médicale dans le 11ème Arrondissement de Paris en 1906," *Bulletin des Syndicats des médecins de France,* (hereinafter: *Bul. des Syn. des Méd. de Fr.),* (July 1901), pp 1090-91; M. Fleury-Ravarin, *Rapport sur les Sécours à domicile à Paris, Conseil superiéur de* l'Assistance publique 1891; Dr. F. Ranse, *Gazette medicale de Paris* S. 7, T. V. N. 48, (Dec. 1888) n.p.

5. *La France médicale* V. 39 N. 18 (April 29, 1892) p 274-75.

6. In 1852 and 1854, the Ministry of the Interior sent out circulairs urging the *Conseils généraux* to organize medical assistance programs. C.S.A.P., Fasc. 22 pp 1-5.

7. Mattew Ramsey, "Medical Power and Popular Medecine: Illegal healers in 19th Century France," *Journal of Social History* (Summer 1977) p 560.

8. "Médecine gratuite en faveur des indigents des campagnes, Tableau 2, fonctionnement en 1887", C.S.A.P., Fasc. 9. pp 49-91. The

percentages reported are based on the thirty-seven departments for which information is available on the functioning of their systems in that year.

9. A study in 1887 showed that the *Loi Roussel* was not being applied at all in twenty-five departments and in most of the rest it was allocated very ineffectual funds. Henri Monod, *Le Concours* V. 10, N. 25 (June 23, 1888) p 294.

10. C.S.A.P. Fasc. 9, Tableau I. "Organisation," pp 4-45.

11. *Ibid.*

12. Jules de Crisenoy, *Questions d'assistance publique traitées dans les Conseils généraux en 1890,* (hereinafter, *Questions)* p 184.

13. de Crisenoy, *Questions,* 1895, pp 200-204; 1898 p 250.

14. de Crisenoy, *Questions,* 1888, pp 149-152; 1890 177-178; 1895, p 190; 1896, p 157.

15. Henri Monod, "Situation des indigents malades dans les communes dépourvues de tout service d'assistance publique", C.S.A.P. Fasc. 29.

16. *Ibid.* pp 32-33.

17. *Ibid.* p 34.

18. *Ibid.* p 36.

19. *Ibid* p 37.

20. *Ibid* p 38-39.

21. *Ibid.*

22. This calculation is based on the forty-eight per cent of the total budget which was derived directly from tax monies. The remainder came from state endowments for public institutions and private endowments. The budget of 1885 was higher than normal for the 1880's due to a special allocation of 2,467,627 francs from the state for victims of the agricultural crisis and 252,537 francs for victims of the cholera epidemics of the previous year; de Crisenoy, "Statistiques des dépenses publique d'Assistance publique en France pendant l'année 1885," *Questions,* 1889, pp 1-5. This was the first government accounting of the funds allocated for assistance in France.

23. Five per cent was allocated for aid to foreigners and repatriation of French nationals: de Crisenoy, *Ibid.*

24. Hautes-Alpes, Ardennes, Aveyron, Corrèze, Corse, Côtes-du-Nord, Doubs, Gironde, Landes, Lot-et-Garonne, Morbihan, Puy-du-Dôme, Basses-Pyrenées, Sarthe, Somme, Vienne, Lozére, Hautes-Pyrenées, all had departmental budgets for public assistance which accounted for 80-100 per cent of the department wide allocations for public assistance. In the overall monies devoted to assistance among the various departments, the assistance council could find no difference between urban and rural departments, and concluded that the amount of monies devoted to assistance were more a function of local customs rather than of wealth: de Crisenoy, *Ibid.* pp 3-23.

25. A number of scholars are currently working ont he problem of social reform in the Second Empire including: Judith Stone, Mary Lynn McDougall, and Lee Shai Weissback.

26. Ibid; *Revue des Etablissements de Bienfaisance* (hereinafter *Rev. des Et. de Bien.*), 1892 p 134.

27. Membership list from the Société de statistique de Paris and same from C.S.A.P. and C.C.H.P.

28. Loua pointed out that seven departments had accounted for one-half of all immigration, Seine, Seine-et-Oise, Loire, Gironde, Pas-de-Calais, Rhône, Meurthe-et-Moselle; Seine absorbed one-fourth of the total immigration. The departments which lost the most population through emigration were Vaucluse, Charente-Inférieure, Gers, Saône-et-Loire, Côtes-du-Nord and Eure; these departments accounted for three-quarters of all emigration; Toussant Loua, "La Dépopulation des Campagnes," *Journal de la Société de la Statistique de Paris*, v. 21 (1880 pp 233-37.

29. l'Abbé Tounissoux, "La Désertion des Campagnes," *Journal de la Société de la Statistique de Paris*, V. 25 (1884) pp 195-204.

30. Ibid.

31. Pierre Joigneaux, "Misére Rurale," *Gazette du Village,* (June 14, 1891), pp 284-285.

32. Stone, op. cit.

33. C.S.A.P., Fasc. 9, p 381.

34. M. Mongeot, *Rapport au Conseil général de la Haute-Marne, enquête de 1872,* C.S.A.P., Fasc. 9 p 382.

35. *Journal Officiel,* N. 75 (March 17, 1891) p 564-55; (see chapter 2.)

36. C.S.A.P., Fasc. 22 p 7; C.S.A.P., Fasc. 9; M. Floquet, "Discours-Séance d'Inauguration, Conseil supérieur de l'Assistance publique," *Le*

Concours, V. 10, N. 25, (June 23, 1888) pp 294-94.

37. C.S.A.P., Fasc. 22; *Rev. des Et. de Bien.,* Jan 1892 pp 133-132. M. Dufaure of the Second Republic had drawn up a comprehensive program of basic assistance, and the right to assistance was written into the constitution of the Second Republic. However, the only solid result of this movement was the law of August 7, 1851 which ostensibly guaranteed hospital care to all French poor.

38. Monod, C.S.A.P., Fasc. 22 p 2.

39. *Rev. des Et. de Bien.,* 1892, pp 136-37.

40. C.S.A.P., Fasc. 22 p 14.

41. C.S.A.P., Fasc. 22 p 3.

42. *Rev. des Et. de Bien.,* 1893 pp 33-38.

43. C.S.A.P., Fasc. 22 p 20.

44. C.S.A.P., Fasc. 22 pp 22-23.

45. "Conseil supérieur de l'Assistance publique séance d'inauguration," *Le Concours,* V. 10, N. 5, (June 23, 1888) pp 294-96.

46. Jacques Léonard, "Les Médecins de l'Ouest aud XIXème siècle," V.III, Chap xvi, note 40.

47. *Le Concours,* V. 13 N. 21 p 241, (May 23, 1891).

48. *Le Concours,* V. 15, n. 45 (Nov. 11, 1893) p 538.

49. C.S.A.P., Fasc. 31, p 1; C.S.A.P., Fasc. 22 p 5.

50. "Allocution de Dr. Lardier," *Bul. des Syn. des Méd. de Fr.,* N. 33, (1889) pp 272-274.

51. "Assemblée générale de la Société du Concours médical, 20 Octobre 1889," *Bulletin des Syndicat des Médecins de France et de l'Union des Syndicats* N. 37, 1889. pp 317-318; C.S.A.P., Fasc. 22 Rapport, II, p 1; Gibert had organized one of the most advanced public health systems while mayor of Le Havre.

52. Dr. Valid, *Le Concours,* V. 9. N. 5 (June 29, 1887) p 56.

53. Dr. Marion, "l'Assistance médicale dans les campagnes," *Le Concours,* V. 12 N. 37 (Sept 13, 1890), p 439.

54. Dr. Lecuyer, "Assistance médicale," *Bulletin des syndicats,* N. 60 (Jan 1892), pp 594-94.

55. "Assistance médicale gratuite," *Rev. des Et. de Bien.,* T. 1895, p 32; Several historians have noted that licensed medical practice met considerable resistance in the nineteenth century from rural people who preferred to use traditional non-licensed practitioners: Jean Pierre Goubert, "l'Art de Guerir, médecine populaire dans la France du 1790," *Annales, Economies, Sociétés and Civilisations,* (Sept.-Oct. 1977); Matthew Ramsey, "Medical Power and Popular Medicine," Illegal Healers in 19th Century France," *Journal of Social History* (Summer 1977).

56. *Le Concours,* V. 12, N. 23 (June 7, 1890) p 271.

57. *Bul. des Syn. des Méd de Fr.,* N. 33, (1889) pp 272-274.

58. M. Lasalle, "Discussion sur proposition de M. le Dr. Gassot au sujet de l'assistance publique," October 1890 Assembly of Le Concours, *Le Concours,* V. 12 N. 47 (Nov. 22, 1890) pp 557.

59. A. Cézilly, *Le Concours* V. 10, N. 9, (May 3, 1888) (n.p.) Dr. Mignen, letter to *Bulletin des syndicats,* N. 33 (n.m. 1889) (n.p.)

60. A. Cézilly, "Commission de l'organisation de l'assistance publique," *Le Concours,* V. 10, N. 14, (April 14, 1888), pp 170-171; V. 10, N. 7, (February 18, 1888) pp 80-81; Dr. Mignen, letter to *Bulletin des syndicats,* N. 33 (n.m. 1889), (n.p.)

61. Dr. Lardier, membre du Conseil supérieur de l'Assistance publique, "l'Assistance médicale dans les campagnes", *Le Concours,* V. 13 N. 12 (Mars 21, 1981) pp 141.

62. A. Gassot, "Le projet de loi sur l'assistance médicale," *Le Concours* V. 12, N. 23 (June 7, 1890) p 271.

63. *Ibid.*

64. A. Gassot, "l'Assistance médicale devant le Sénat, *Le Concours,* V. 15 N. 14, (April 8, 1893) n.p.; A. Cézilly, "l'Assistance médicale dans toute la France," *Le Concours* V. 12 N. 22 (May 31, 1890) n.p.

65. A. Cézilly and L. Porsons, *Le Concours,* V. 15 N. 12 (March 25, 1893) pp 140-141.

66. Gassot, V. 12, N. 47, (Nov. 22, 1890) pp 556-557.

67. Dr. Lardier, "l'Assistance médicale dans les campagnes," *Le Concours,* (March 21, 1891) p 141; Gassot was not placated by Lardier's reassurances and continued to warn his fellow doctors of the dangers of the spread of dispensaries under the medical assistance program, however his fears were not realized.

68. C.S.A.P., Fasc. 9, Tableau I; George Weisz, "The Politics of Medical Professionalization in France 1845-1848," *Journal of Social History,* V. 12 N. 1 (Fall 1978).

69. *Le Concours,* V. 14, N. 30, (July 23, 1892) pp 350-59.

70. Paul Brouardel, *De l'Exercise et de l'Enseignement de la médecine,* 1873, n.p.

71. "l'Assistance médicale dans de 11ème Arrondissement de Paris en 1900," *Bulletin des syndicats des Médecins de France,* July 1901, pp 1090-1091; M. Fleury-Ravarin, *Rapport sur les sécours à Domicile à Paris à Conseil supérieur de l'Assistance publique,* 1891; Dr. F. Ranse, *Gazette médicale de Paris,* S. 7, T.V., N.48, (Dec., 1888, p 843

72. C.S.A.P., Fasc. 9. Tableau II; In 1896 Medical Assistance was still not functioning in a large part of the Vosges: de Crisenoy, *Question.,* 1896 pp 172-173.

73. Dr. Porsons, "Assistance médicale gratuite," *Bulletin des Syndicats des Médecins de France* N. 36, 1889, p 301; Dr. Mignen, op. cit., N. 33, 1889 n.p.; *Lyon médical,* No 41, (Oct 8, 1893) pp 210-212; *Le Concours,* V. 10, N. 7 (Feb. 18, 1888), pp 80-82; V. 10, N. 10 (April 21, 1888), pp 182-183; V. 13, N. 13 (March 21, 1891) p 141; V. 12 N. 37, (Sept 13, 1890), p 439; V. 14 N. 26, (June 25, 1892) pp 308-310; V. 14, N. 27, (July 2, 1892) pp 319-321.

74. *Le Concours,* V. 13 N. 47 (Sept 21, 1891) pp 554-557.

75. Dr. Porsons, "Projet de reglement de service gratuit de l'assistance médicale et pharmaceutique des indigents du département de la Loire-

Inférieure," *Le Concours,* V. 14, N. 27 (July 2, 1892) pp 319-321.

76. Dr. Gassot, "À M. le Dr. Porson," *Le Concours,* V. 14, N. 27 (July 2, 1892) pp 321-22.

77. *Le Concours* V. 10 N. 16 (April 21, 1888) pp 182-83.

78. *Le Concours,* V. 10, N. 16 (April 21, 1888) pp 182-83; the Medical Assistance quarrels in Seine-et-Oise are described in more detail in the following chapter.

79. C.S.A.P., "Rapport à Monsieur le Président du Conseil, Ministre de l'Intérieur et des Cultes concernant l'execution pendant les années 1897, 1898, et 1899 de la Loi de 15 Juillet 1893 sur l'Assistance médicale gratuite," Fasc. 92, pp 13-15.

80. Dr. Mignen, "Assistance médicale gratuite," *Bul. des Syn. des Med. dr Fr.,* N. 33 (1889).

81. de Crisenoy, *Questions,* 1895 pp 219-220.

82. see following chapter.

83. de Crisenoy, *Questions* 1888 n.p.; 1895 pp 707-08; 1896 p 169.

84. RCC V. 18, (1888) p 207.

85. Henri Monod, Directeur de l'Assistance publique, letter to Charles Floquet, Ministére de l'Intérieur, Paris, 10 June 1888, printed in C.S.A.P., Fasc. 22.

86. C.S.A.P., Fasc. 22 p 15.

87. *Ibid* pp 16-17.

88. C.S.A.P., Fasc. 9; Fasc. 22.

89. See chapter 4.

90. C.S.A.P., Fasc. 22, pp 28-29.

91. C.S.A.P., Fasc. 22, pp 1-5.

92. *Ibid.*

93. This statistic might reflected the fact that in spite of the lack of national legislation, much of urban France had a more extensive system of assistance than either Britain or Germany at the end of the nineteenth century.

94. C.S.A.P., Fasc. 22, pp 6-15.

95. *Ibid.* p 30.

96. *Ibid* pp 33-35.

97. The assistance council echoed a growing state concern with the increase numbers of government bureaucrats. Thus the state at this time was just beginning to echo a fear which Doctors had had for a long time.

98. *Le Concours,* V. 14 N. 4, (Jan 23, 1892) p 47. In 1887 most communes in the Vosges refused to participate in the system, as Dreyfus-Brisac himself noted; C.S.A.P., Fascs 92, pp 11-13. In 1895 the medical assistance system in Vosges was still not functioning in a large part of the department; de Crisenoy, *Questions,* 1896 pp 172-73. Bosges reported statistics in 1887 which indicate that the department was spending 2.97 francs per indigent treated. In that same year, the other Landais systems in operation had an average cost of 15.13 francs per

indigent treated, and all systems together averaged 9.50 francs per indigent: C.S.A.P., Fascs 9, Tableau II. pp 48-90. The Landais systems of 1899 had an average cost of 18.17 francs per indigent treated; *Le Concours,* V. 10, N. 16 (April 211, 1888) pp 182-83. The very low expenditures reported in Vosges indicate that the system was working badly; at these rates doctors could not have been paid by the visit, unless they saw each patient only once and prescribed no medications. Nevertheless, Dreyfus-Brisac used the Vosges as his model in claiming that the Landais system was as efficient as the Cantonal in reaching needy indigents and keeping costs down. In his other model, Loire the system in operation was, as we have seen, more like the Cantonal.

99. C.S.A.P., Fasc., 9.

100. *Ibid.*

101. Levasseur.

102. de Crisenoy, *Questions,* 1895 pp 184-187; 1898 p 70; 1899 p 113.

103. de Crisenoy, *Questions,* 1889, p 187.

104. de Crisenoy *Questions,* 1888 p 139.

105. *Ibid.*

106. *Gazette hebd. de Bordeaux,* V. 12 N. 8, (Feb. 22, 1891) p 94.

107. Foucault, op. cit.; Alan Forrest, "La Révolution et les hôpitaux dans le département de la Gironde," *Annales du Midi* T. 86, N. 119, pp 381; Muriel Jeorger, "La Structure hospitaliére de la France sous l'ancien régime," *A.E.S.C.,* (Sept.-Oct. 1977) pp 1025-1049.

108. C.S.A.P., Fasc. 22.

109. H. Monod, "l'Assistance médicale gratuite en 1895," *Rev. des Et. de Bien.*, 1896 p 209; de Crisenoy, 1895 p 200.

110. Pierre Joigneaux, "l'Assistance publique dans les campagnes," *Gazette du Village*, v. 25, n. 5 (Jan 22, 1888, p 53;

111. *Ibid.*

112. de Crisenoy, *Questions,* 1893, pp 191-192.

113. "Rapport de M. Gueneau", de Crisenoy, *Questions,* 1889, p 187.

114. Dr. Saloman, "Rapport à la Congrés d'Assistance familiale sur l'Assistance médicale en famille à la campagne," *Bulletin official de l'Union des Syndicats médicaux de France* Jan. 20 1902.

115. de Crisenoy, *Questions,* 1889, p 187; This comment illustrates the lingering fear of hospitals because of their association with the hôpitaux généraux.

116. C.S.A.P., Fasc. 29, 1890 pp 2-3.

117. C.S.A.P., session, Feb. 1890, C.S.A.P.; Fasc. 31, p 28-29.

118. de Crisenoy, *Questions,* 1888, p 150, 133.

119. *Ibid.*

120. *C.S.A.P., Séance, Feb. 1890,* pp 36-28.

121. C.S.A.P., Fasc. 9, Tableaux I and II; A Mann-Whitney analysis of central tendancy was used due to small sample size, significance was accepted at the $<.05$ level. Corse was left out of the sample because medical care in that department reflected non-French traditions and

officiers de santé dominated medical care. The Vosges was also left out for reasons discussed earlier in the chapter. In determining the systems the criteria of method of payment was used. This meant the inclusion of one department as having the Landais system where payment was made by visit but doctors were appointed, and the inclusion of one department as cantonal where in some communes all doctors were allowed to participate if they so chose.

122. *Ibid.*

123. *Ibid.*

124. *Ibid.*

CHAPTER V

THE IMPACT OF THE MEDICAL ASSISTANCE LAW,

1893-1902

The physicians' Union movement and the Public Assistance Council were remarkably successful in promoting the Landais system of medical assistance. Before the 1893 law went into effect, only thirteen per cent of those departments with medical assistance programs had instituted the Landais system; by 1899 fifteen-seven per cent of departments used this system. [1] Before 1893, sixty-five per cent of the departments had used the cantonal system for medical assistance; by 1899 only sixteen per cent still used that system. The remaining departments had mixed systems, twenty-seven per cent in 1899 and twenty-two per cent before 1893 (see Table IV-1 and Table V-1). [2] This rapid and widespread substitution of the Landais system for cantonal medical assistance was the result of local syndicats taking up the program of arguments and lobbying that the Union of Syndicats and the society, Le Concours, had developed between 1888 and 1892. In many cases, however, the task of the local syndicats was not easy. Many local officials (departmental councilors, prefects and mayors) were not receptive towards the idea of medical assistance, nor were they anxious to further the professional goals inherent in the Union's plan for the enactment of the Medical Assistance Law.

Many struggles, often bitter and lengthy ones, took place between doctors and local officials over the enactment of the Medical Assistance Law. Local officials were often quite skeptical of the necessity and the feasibility of the law. Doctors, on the other hand, complained about the way which departments applied the Medical Assistance Law, charging departmental officials with evasion. The doctors also objected to the fees they were paid under the programs and the way in which lists of eligible indigents were made up. In many departments the physicians' syndicats were well prepared before the Medical Assistance Law was passed to force the Landais system upon their departmental council. In the years after 1893, the local doctors' syndicats worked assiduously against cantonal (circumscription) systems where they still existed. [3] By the end of the first decade of national medical assistance, however, many of the Landais systems had run into financial trouble. Departmental officials, alarmed over high expenses, began to attempt to modify their programs away from the Landais model. Throughout this era, doctors in many areas of the nation were militant in their insistence on the Landais system and did not hesitate to threaten non-cooperation or in some cases to actually strike against systems they opposed. This chapter will survey the medical assistance programs in the departments, focusing on the role of the local physicians syndicats in their development. The chapter is based upon information gathered for fifty-five departments, about 63% of the total.

The conflicts between doctors and local officials were not the only obstacles to medical assistance. In some departments undersupply of practitioners was a great barrier to creating medical assistance programs. In the department of Pyrenées-Orientales officials found it difficult to create an organization because so many communes in mountainous areas were without doctors, pharmacists or *officiers de santé*. In the arrondissement of Prades, for example, four cantons were without a single doctor. Other cantons were regularly cut off in the winter from access to practitioners. The department attempted to get extra funds from the state to finance the transfer of physicians from other departments in the area which were oversupplied with practitioners. When the state refused, a departmental councilor noted bitterly that the French government spent more in his department on veterinary services than medical care for its human population. [4]

The case of Haute-Loire illustrates the problems encountered in establishing a medical assistance program in a department with an extreme variation in the density of practitioners per population. Overall the department's ratio of practitioners to population was very low: 1/6723 in 1896. But the cities were well supplied with doctors. The city of Le Puy had one doctor for every 2030 people and the city of Brioude had one for every 714. In the rural cantons it was another story. In the cantons of the arrondissement of Le Puy, outside of the city of Le Puy and its suburban area, there were 18,285 people for every doctor. In the arrondissements of Brioude and Yssingeaux there were 4555 and 7000 residents for every doctor, respectively. In the department as a whole there were a total of nine cantons of 77,000 total population without any practitioners at all. [5]

In April 1895 the department of Haute-Loire attempted to establish a cantonal type system of medical assistance which paid stipends of one thousand francs a year to doctors. However, only two communes in the department agreed to cooperate. Most of the other communes said that there were not enough doctors to establish a system. The departmental council then proposed a system of one dispensary in each canton, where visiting doctors would hold specified office hours and where medicines and supplies would be on hand. Doctors outside of Le Puy and the arrondissement of Brioude agreed to work for two days a month at the dispensaries. The doctors of Le Puy demanded and got their duties curtailed to one day a month. In the arrondissement of Brioude the doctors refused to cooperate at all. In 1898 the departmental physicians' syndicat, led by the doctors of Brioude, forced the department to abandon the dispensaries altogether and institute the Landais system. [6] In the arrondissement of Brioude, and the suburban area around Le Puy, where the density of doctors was high, the Landais system was feasible and duly enacted. In the rest of the department, however, the Landais system could not function, and medical assistance was not put into effect. Thus doctors organized in the urban areas succeeded in preventing the enactment of the only sort of medical assistance, dispensary care, which might have brought medical care to the rural areas of the department.

Ironically, although medical assistance was sold to the legislature as a program to bring licensed medical care to rural France, this was not the guiding principle in establishing medical assistance systems. Rather it was the professional needs of doctors in areas oversupplied with practitioners which governed the establishment of systems. The doctors' main concern was to use medical assistance to control competition for clients and expand clienteles in areas with high physician density. The Landais system met these concerns. The systems which could have had immediate impact in relocating doctors, the cantonal and dispensary systems, were everywhere opposed by doctors.

The Medical Assistance Law sparked the founding of doctors' syndicats in a number of departments and reactivated syndicats which had been founded between 1888 and 1893. It signaled the beginning of an era of unprecedented activism among the physicians' syndicats which then spread from medical assistance to other issues. In many departments the departmental councils found its doctors well prepared in advance of the law to force the adoption of the Landais system. In Cantal, for example, the council adopted a circumscription system in 1894 only to discover that the physicians' syndicat immediately refused to participate. The following year the council bowed to the doctors and adopted the Landais system. [7] Doctors in Marne profited from the presence of Dr. Henrot on the C.S.A.P. (National Public Assistance Council) subcommittee on medical assistance. Henrot kept the Marne syndicat well informed on the law's progress in Paris and the syndicat in turn used his prestige to promote the Landais system in the department. In

Marne, as in many other departments, medical assistance and the *Loi Chevandier* were connected. At Henrot's urging, the doctors' syndicat scheduled a series of meetings with Senators, Deputies and departmental officials to lobby in favor of the two bills and the Landais system. [8] A similar sequence of events took place between the physicians' syndicats and departmental councils of Puy-de-Dôme and Charente-Inférieure. [9]

The case of Seine-et-Oise illustrates the parameters of the conflict over medical assistance in a department where doctors were well organized and the bureaucratic medical establishment was also well entrenched. Seine-et-Oise, one of the most populous departments in the nation, was a hotbed of early Union activity on the part of doctors (see Chapter I). The medical syndicat of the arrondissement of Versailles (Seine-de-Oise) was founded in 1887 for the purpose of making an impact upon the organization of medical assistance in the department. The syndicat's founder was Dr. Fourmestreaux, one of the co-founders of the *Union des Syndicats médicaux de France* (and President of the Union) and a departmental councilor in Seine-et-Oise. Dr. Fourmestreaux's local syndicat covered the suburban area of the arrondissement of Versailles (doctors practicing in the city of Versailles had their own separate syndicat.) Fourmestreaux's suburban syndicat included two-thirds of the doctors practicing in that area. In 1889 he united all the local syndicats in the department into a union of Seine-et-Oise doctors, including the local syndicats in the city of Versailles, Mantes, Pontoise, Rambouillet, Corbeil, as well as Fourmestraux's own local. [10]

Seine-et-Oise had an extensive hospital network. In the mid-1880s the departmental council planned to create a medical assistance system based on hospital care with the addition of several new hospitals. However, after extensive lobbying by syndicat doctors, this idea was pushed aside and medical assistance was reorganized in 1888 under a Landais program. Fourmestreaux and two other members of the Versailles arrondissement syndicat, Drs. Jeanne and Mignon were able to get the departmental budget for medical assistance raised from 19,000 to 40,000 francs. Fees were 2.50 francs per visit with extra payment for travel over two kilometers. These payments were in keeping with the Union campaign to wipe out the tradition of one franc per visit which was common in rural practice. [11]

After having seen the enactment of the Landais system in their department, the Seine-et-Oise syndicat turned its attention to enforcing the commune's compliance with that system. In 1890 the syndicat invited Cézilly to a meeting with the Senators and Deputies of the department. At this meeting doctors tried to convince their legislators to pressure the communes to comply with the Landais system, which about one third of the department's communes refused to accept. [12] Ironically, in this heartland of the Union movement, the medical assistance program functioned very poorly. By 1899 the department had switched over to payment by stipend while maintaining free choice of doctors and patients. The funds spent on the system were the lowest in France, 3.0 francs per indigent as compared to a national average of 16.3, indicating that the program was virtually non-functional. [13] In

1900 the syndicat notified the department prefect that it intended to strike against several communes where the municipal government refused to participate in the system. [14] In that year the Public Assistance Council reported that the system was still not operating in accordance with the law and substantial areas of the department were not participating. The statistics on the functioning of the system in 1900 indicate that a limited number of the department's poor were being reached by the system. [15]

The department of Vienne was the location of another concerted effort by syndicat doctors to organize their favored form of medical assistance. The program in Vienne was greatly publicized in the pages of Le Concours as a good example of the Landais system. Two physicians' syndicats in Vienne had launched a campaign in the departmental council against "médecins-fonctionnaires" and the cantonal systems which existed in some areas of the department. The syndicats painted a dismal picture of the functioning of medical assistance in these areas. They succeeded in impressing their views on a commission of the departmental council which organized a new system in 1888. The commission stated that there two kinds of medicine being practiced in Vienne, "...official medicine" and "free medicine." Far from being an honor, the commission noted that the title of médecin fonctionnaire "puts an intolerable work load on the cantonal doctor for which he is poorly compensated, but worst of all he suffers from a moral decline and finds his position in society to be denigrated." [16] The commission advocated the institution of the Landais system but by 1889 only 188 of

300 communes were participating; the rest refused to comply. [17]

Disgruntled communal officials in Vienne complained about the high costs and blamed the poor and doctors for abusing prescriptions. [18] Dr. Guillon of the Vienne syndicat, writing in the pages of *Le Concours,* blamed the high costs on mayors and their alleged negligence in controlling the program. [19] The department council finally decided that other forms of aid were more critical to the department's poor, especially with the agricultural crisis of 1891-1892. The council transferred funds from the medical assistance program in order to finance a system of *ateliers de charité* (workshops and welfare centers.) The council was very critical of its medical assistance system, and joined the departmental councils of Tarn and Eure in demanding modification of the law to enable the departments to return to the system they had had in effect before 1889. In the case of Vienne, the pre-1893 system was a cantonal program which was voluntary on the part of the communes. [20]

In the densely populated departments Rhône and Gironde, doctors' syndicats found strong opposition to medical assistance among members of local government. In the Rhône the syndicat doctors were thoroughly triumphant in enforcing their views on the department. In the Gironde doctors failed to maintain a department-wide Landais system, but they succeeded in obtaining a tariff schedule of added fees for surgery and special care under the medical assistance program.

In the department of Rhône bureaucratic medical care began in 1867 with the establishment of the *Service sanitaire* The service operated under the secretary general of police and consisted of regular medical examinations of prositutes for evidence of venereal disease. In 1878 the departmental council looked into the possibility of creating a department-wide system of medical assistance but after a survey found only seventy-two communes to be interested in such a program. In 1882 the physician-mayor of Lyon, Dr. Gailleton, who was also on the C.S.A.P. subcommittee on medical assistance, organized a *bureau de bienfaisance* which was aimed in part at providing medical assistance for the indigents of the city. [21]

To staff the *bureau de bienfaisance,* eighteen doctors were nominated and each given responsibility for care in a particular part of the city for a yearly stipend of 2000 francs. [22] When it became a question of providing similar services to the indigents of the countryside, the departmental council was quite resistant. In 1895 the council sent off a protest to the *Conseil d'Etat* over the prerogative given to the Ministry of the Interior to require the departments to institute taxes to support medical assistance. [23] Some of the departmental councilors questioned the effectiveness of professional medical care and the usefulness of promoting a program which would increase the number of doctors in the countryside: "...if medical assistance takes the form of consultations by doctors we will have more doctors then we need. In our areas the fewer the doctors, the better we feel!" Several other councilors expressed the view that if medical assistance was enacted its funds should be used to pay unlicensed practitioners as well. [24]

As was the case in so many departments, the medical assistance issue brought a tremendous increase in the membership and activities of the Rhône medical syndicat. [25] In 1895, after much pressure from the syndicat, the department prefect appointed a commission to study medical assistance. The president of the Rhône medical syndicat was named to the commission along with six doctors from the department council; three other members were pharmacists and there were two non-medical departmental councilors. [26] In the commission's report the views of the syndicat were well represented. For two years the syndicat members, mainly rural doctors, had argued over the best means of organizing the system. Ultimately a majority of doctors were convinced of the benefits of the Landais system and the commission adopted it along with a fee schedule promoted by the syndicat. The commission defended its adoption of these measures by explaining that its main goal was to create a system which would "...ménager la dignité du corps médical." [27] The recommendations of the Rhône medical assistance commission were enacted, but the departmental councilors subsequently complained a great deal about the program in action. The councilors pointed out that because the fee schedule called for added payments to doctors for travel over two kilometers, doctors in some areas received higher fees for caring for indigents that they did for their regular clients. In the town of Villechenève, which had no doctor in residence, the town council was forced to pay twelve francs per indigent to the doctor who had been traveling there regularly anyway. This doctor, it was reported, received only six francs from his regular paying clients in Villechèneve. The town council petitioned to the departmental council for dispensation from the departmental fee scheduled and asked to deal directly with the doctor themselves. This was granted over the protests of several doctors who were members of the departmental council. Dr. Lasale, who voiced the Syndicat position in the council, objected that this growing tendency to grant dispensations to various communes was dangerous because in creating their own medical assistance systems, the communes typically took away the freedom of the indigents to choose their own doctor. Another councilor responded that urban indigents in Lyon had no such right. He might well have added that indigents living in town like Villechenève in reality had no alternatives regardless of the system in effect, because only one doctor visited their commune. [28]

The Rhône syndicat continued to keep a close watch on the functioning of medical assistance, particularly through Dr. Lasalle. The syndicat urged its members to refuse to deal individually with communes, apparently with some effectiveness. The commune of Propiéres was unable to find a Rhône doctor who would accept their medical assistance terms and began to negotiate with a doctor from neighboring Saône-et-Loire. Several other communes followed this example, making deals with doctors in Saône-et-Loire and Loire. The syndicat protested to doctors in those two departments and requested that the syndicats there pressure their fellow doctors to back out of any arrangements they had made with the Rhône communes. In addition to competition from the doctors of neighboring departments, the Rhône doctors noted that in dealing directly with local communities they also faced competition from illegal practitioners for medical assistance monies. [29]

The Rhône syndicat succeeded in destroying a community medical program in the commune of Chossy-les-Mines. As a result of a bequest, the commune had decided to hire both a doctor and pharmacists and provide them with homes and annual salaries. They would then be expected to treat all the residents of the commune with no additional charges. In 1902 the syndicat saw to it that this program was discontinued and replaced with the Landais system for indigents only. [30] The syndicat monitored communes which had neglected to make up lists of indigents or had put too few indigents on the lists. The syndicat pressured the department and communes to require the participation of doctors in deciding who would be eligible for medical assistance. In 1902 the syndicat also succeeded in having a surgery and obstetrical fee schedule attached to the system. [31]

The general political influence of the Rhône syndicat increased as a result of its organization to control medical assistance. Its influence was enhanced by close relationship with other doctors in political positions such as Dr. Gailleton, and Dr.-Professeur Augagnieu who was elected major of Lyon in 1902. The syndicat used its influence in other issues as well. For instance, in 1902 the syndicat successfully blocked a program initiated by the prefect of the Rhône to admit a special category of entrants, without the classical baccalaureate into the *Ecole de médecine*. The prefect had hoped that his move would solve the serious problem of undersupply of practitioners in the rural areas of Rhône. The syndicat argued that this would amount to recreating the *officiers de santé*. [32]

The Gironde was another area of intense activity over medical assistance. In 1889, 358 doctors in the department organized to promote free medical care in anticipation of the Medical Assistance Law. The stated purpose was to spread free care to all of the department based on the Landais system. The syndicat publicized several deaths of indigents due to lack of care which they blamed upon unconcerned mayors. The doctors pursuaded the department to adopt the Landais system in 1894, in spite of considerable opposition from some members of the departmental council who maintained that it was simply not true that indigents were dying for lack of medical care. [33]

By 1896 the animosity on the Gironde council had worsened. One member advocated abolishing the Landais system and petitioning the national legislature to abrogate the 1893 law. The council was alarmed over expenses; it was reported that communes around Bordeaux which before the law had spent about 2,500 francs per year on the average to care for indigents were now spending 8,000 and their services to indigents were no better. M. Bertin of the commune of Cauderon reported that 138 indigents there had been cared for in 1895 at an expense of 8,504 francs. In previous years roughly the same number had been cared for at about half the cost. The councilors blamed abuses by doctors and indigents for these problems. Ultimately they abolished the Landais system and instead allowed the communes to each deal directly with local doctors. [34]

In spite of this setback, the Gironde physicians' syndicat went on to create a new aspect of state medicine which compensated in part for their failure to maintain the Landais system. The syndicat developed a surgical and obstetric fee schedule which became known as the *Tarif Girondin*. The tariff provided for added payments under medical assistance for these services. This fee schedule took on added importance when it was adopted by the national government for the Law on Work Accidents of 1898 which provided that employers would be responsible for their employees' medical expenses in the care of job-related injuries. Doctors in the Gironde and throughout the nation objected that worker-clients were worth more in fees than indigents, and in 1903 a new tariff schedule was created reflecting the higher fees habitually charged workers. This new *Tarif-Girondin* stipulated a twenty-five per cent reduction when used for fees charged for indigent care under medical assistance. The *Tarif-Girondin* received wide publicity throughout the country, was promoted by syndicats all over and adopted in many departments for the Medical Assistance and Work Accidents Laws. [35]

Although doctors' syndicats were generally well prepared and organized to deal with the implementation of the Medical Assistance Law, they frequently ran up against insurmountable obstacles created by the animosities of local officials. The attitudes of local officials towards doctors and medical assistance was often a marked contrast to that of the legislators and bureaucrats of the state. Throughout the country departmental councilors expressed hostility and anger at being forced to institute medical assistance. Sometimes they objected to the general idea of state medical assistance for indigents; at other times they objected to the principle of the state, in effect, supporting doctors. They also criticized the Landais system, especially in departments where there had been a cantonal system in use. In Sarthe, where medical assistance had been in operation since the 1850s as an addition to an extensive program for *enfants assistés,* the departmental council objected to the efforts of the doctors' syndicat to force the creation of the Landais system. The head of the medical assistance commission noted, "It is evident that some doctors here believe that a new situation has been created which must translate into new sacrifices on the part of the collectivity, in new payments for their services," [36] In some departments this opposition was strong enough to delay the initiation of medical assistance, and in a few cases, the departmental government refused to set up a department wide organization for medical assistance but rather simply created a budget and left it up to the communes to deal with doctors. By the late 1890s the departments of Pas-de-Calais, Mayenne, Lot-et-Garonne and Hautes-Pyrenées still refused outright to apply the law of 1893. Eventually, the *Conseil d'Etat* was forced to intervene in some of these cases. [37] Several departmental councils passed resolutions demanding the law be revised so that it was less binding upon the local governments. [38]

Local officials and even some doctors were afraid of the implications of making assistance obligatory. Dr. Fayel, a member of the departmental council of Calvados and president of the local branch of the *Association Générale des Médecins français* warned of

"the difficulties created by the obligation dictated by the law. Charity cannot be decreed, it is practiced freely and it disappears when obligation begins." [39]

But Fayel argued that if medical assistance was made obligatory upon doctors then they should be compensated according to the fees they normally earned. Local officials also expressed concern over the possible effects of medical assistance upon family cohesiveness. In Indre-et-Loire the inspector of medical assistance reassured the departmental council that the goal was not to substitute assistance for the natural duties of the family but rather to use it to promote family cohesiveness. [40]

Resistance to medical assistance came from communal authorities as well. Some mayors attempted to avoid the issue by not enlisting indigents; other mayors maintained that all their residents were in need of aid to pay for medical care. [41] Doctors alternatively complained that mayors were taking too much authority upon themselves in limiting who would be cared for and when, or that mayors were neglecting the system, or were allowing too many enrollments. [42] In several departments the number of non-participating communes was still quite large several years after departmental medical assistance programs had been put into effect. In the Vosges thirty per cent of the communes did not take part in the program in 1896, at least seven years after it had purportedly been created. [43] In the Jura, in 1898, the system was not functioning in about forty per cent of the communes. [44] In 1899 about seven per cent of all communes in France did not participate in their departmental medical assistance programs, according to the figures reported to the Public Assistance Council. This figure probably under-represented the actual number of communes not taking part in the programs since it was based upon the communes creating a medical assistance budget, not on whether they actually made lists and awarded aid. [45]

The above survey has shown that struggles over medical assistance were confined to no particular area. Rather the conflicts of physicians' syndicats and local government accompanied medical assistance in the nation as a whole, becoming critical where doctors were well organized. The issues upon which doctors insisted were also consistent: the Landais system as the only method of instituting medical assistance; controls on the formation of lists of eligible indigents; and the participation of local doctors in running the system.

The struggles over medical assistance were particularly intense in the area of the Garonne Basin. Here the rate of practitioners to population was the highest of all regions in France and competition for clients seems to have been a major issue. In 1896, in response to the medical assistance issue, doctors' syndicats in this area created the *Fédération des Médecins du Sud-Quest,* centered in Toulouse (Haute-Garonne), which also included syndicats in Ariège, Aude, Aveyron, Gers, Lot-et-Garonne, Hautes-Pyrenées, Pyrenées-Orientales, Tarn, and Tarn-et-Garonne. Membership numbers in these departmental syndicats were impressive. In 1897 the Haute-Garonne syndicat had 132 members, Hautes-Pyrenées 102, and Tarn 72; by 1901 the Haute-Garonne syndicat had grown to 150. [46]

The syndicat of Haute-Garonne, which organized the local federation, was the leader in medical assistance activism. The syndicat struggled intensely with the departmental government over medical assistance. Haute-Garonne doctors felt they were in a poor bargaining position because their department had one of the highest rates of doctors per population in the nation. They pointed out that the medical faculties at Toulouse and Montpellier produced scores of new doctors each year, many of whom were anxious to stay and practice in this attractive and relatively prosperous region. The doctors sought to counter the ill effects of this situation under the aggressive leadership of Dr. Lucien Dore, who was the Auguste Cézilly of the south. After founding the Haute-Garonne syndicat, Dore created *La Fédération Médicale de la Sud-Ouest* and began publication of a newsletter for the organization. The federation fostered an aggressive front of doctors in all the departments of the area. [47]

Dore's main enemy over medical assistance was Jean Bepmale, an important politician of the radical party and a departmental councilor of Haute-Garonne who was the watchdog of public assistance. Under Bepmale's domination, the departmental council was highly resistant to the Landais system. [48] Haute-Garonne adopted its first medical assistance program in 1895 under a circumscription system. In 1896, after numerous complaints by doctors, the department experimented with payment by visit. In several cantons the "Remy" system was put into effect, whereby the cantons were given a set budget for doctors' fees which they divided among all their participating doctors according to the number of visits they made to indigent patients. In twenty communes a true Landais system was tried out. The result of these two experiments was that the costs for medical assistance increased from 78,000 francs in 1895 to 102,974 in 1896. Mayors complained that doctors were guilty of over-prescribing under both the Landais and Remy systems. The mayors pointed out that the indigents, like all patients, tended to favor doctors who prescribed the most; doctors competing for indigent patronage were drawn into fulfilling their patients' expectations. The results were bills to medical assistance such as was submitted by the pharmacist of one commune, 200 francs worth of saccharine for a diabetic indigent during a five month period. Dore argued to the departmental council that such abuses could be solved by regulations on prescriptions but the council was generally ill disposed toward these experiments with the Remy and Landais systems. [49]

In 1899 after having pushed the Landais system unsuccessfully, the Haute-Garonne syndicat decided to make a comprehensive survey of the medical assistance views of doctors in the department. They discovered that the pro-Landais position of the local syndicat did not reflect the wishes of the majority of practitioners in the department. Sixty-six of 156 doctors and *officiers de santé* in the department responded to the inquiry: forty-four responded in favor of stipends and only twenty-two in favor of payment by visit. There was a general geographical split between the arrondissement of Saint-Gaudens and the arrondissements of Toulouse, Muret and Villefranche. Saint-Gaudens doctors preferred stipends and set circumscriptions. This corresponded to their normal relationships with their clients in the Southern part of the department, where, according to Dore, doctors preserved the "old custom" of caring for client-families on the basis of a yearly fee set in advance upon the family's ability to pay rather than services rendered. The doctors of this area claimed this was a way of preserving both their dignity and their close relationship with their client-families. It also allowed them to tailor their fees to the actual wealth and status of the families. They argued that payment by visit in fact placed hardships on families at the time when they could least afford it especailly if one of the breadwinners was ill. For the doctors, this practice assured them of a steady, if modest, income, and the lack of competition kept new doctors out, particularly advantageous given the steady number of new doctors produced each year by the two faculties of medicine in the area. Rather than despising the position of *médecin-fonctionnaire*, doctors in Saint-Gaudens sought the position of "medecin d'assistance," and reported that the status associated with the title was absolutely necessary in maintaining a clientele. [50] Thus the Saint-Gaudens doctors supported everything the Union was fighting against: pre-paid medical care and support for *médecin-fonctionnaires*.

In the area around Toulouse and on the "Plaine" (roughly, the arrondissements of Muret and Villefranche) the situation was quite different. In these areas competition for clients was intense and payment by visit was the favored system. The syndicat movement was also concentrated in this area. In 1899, faced with the opposition of Saint-Gaudens doctors, Dore was forced to abandon the demand for the

Landais system and the syndicat decided to promote a revision of the 1897 system which would allow for free choice of doctors by clients in a territorial circumscription which would be drawn in such a way as to replicate each doctor's current practice. This system was adopted and put into effect in 1900, but in 1901 the doctors of Muret went on strike against the system, still hoping to obtain the Landais system. Bepmale continued to complain about "...le ton imperatif" of the doctors and political struggles over medical assistance continued through 1914. [51]

In several other departments in the area covered by Dore's southern federation, doctors carried out strikes in favor of the Landais system; some were successful and others were not. With the encouragement of the federation, the doctors' syndicat of Ariège took more drastic action than their leaders in Toulouse. In 1894 the departmental council of Ariège voted in a circumscription system with doctors' yearly stipends fixed at 10 centimes per inhabitant. The syndicat complained that because they were taxed on the basis of total inhabitants rather than indigents, communes were enlisting too many of their residents as eligible for medical assistnce. On January 10, 1899, syndicat doctors went on strike against medical assistance. Of the sixty-five doctors enrolled in the system, fifty-four refused to serve. [52] The syndicat demanded that it be allowed to draw up the circumscriptions, which in effect meant that the syndicat would control who practiced under medical assistance. They also demanded that the number of eligible indigents be considerably reduced and extra payments be made on the basis of travel to indigents' homes. The syndicat also complained that although their

Senator, M. Delpech, had been their "energetic defender," the three doctors on the departmental council were not helping them at all. [53] The strike continued through the end of 1900.

In both Hautes-Pyrenées and Aveyron doctors also syndicalized and went on strike against the medical assistance system adopted by their departmental council. As in Ariège, the doctors' syndicat of Aveyron complained that although there were 10 doctor-members on their departmental council, their political brothers gave them no support on medical assistance. When directly criticized for this, the doctor-councilors explained to the syndicat they were elected to serve the interests of their communes rather than their fellow doctors. [54]

The Aveyron syndicat was particularly incensed that the original planning commission for medical assistance had advocated the Landais system only to have it rejected by the departmental council. In November of 1897, the doctors of Rodez wrote to the prefect to protest the insults they had received from one councilor in the discussions over medical assistance and to announce a plan to strike as of January 1, 1898 if the Landais system was not adopted. [55]

In 1895 the Hautes-Pyrenées departmental council adopted a system under which rural doctors were to be paid five francs per indigent family per year, with the families given the prerogative to choose their physician. In direct response, ninety-six of the department's 125 doctors syndicalized in 1897 and joined La Fédération médicale. [56] In November of 1898 the syndicat notified the council that they would go on strike if the Landais system was not substituted. [57] In 1899 the syndicat settled for a partial victory. The council agreed to a system whereby all doctors were eligible to participate and were to be paid a yearly stipend based upon the number of indigents they served, supplemented by a travel fee based upon distances traveled to visit their indigent clients. [58]

The longest struggle over the insitution of medical assistance took place in Lot-et-Garonne, another department where the doctors' syndicat was a member of the southern federation. This department was the last in the nation to institute a medical assistance program. It took threats of legal action from the National Public Assistance Council and a strike threat from the local doctors syndicat to force the departmental council to act. A medical assistance system was formally adopted in 1895, but througout its next five sessions the council refused to vote any funds. [59] Some councilors protested the expenses while others claimed that the law would impose too much structure on charity which was already more than adequate in the department. One councilor told the Public Assistance Council that such a law was not needed in Lot-et-Garonne; no indigents had ever died for lack of medical care. In October of 1899 the council adopted a motion requesting that the national legislature amend the medical assistance law so that the departments would have more flexibility in dealing with the situations in individual communes. In spite of the councilors' excuses, the syndicat claimed that the main reason for the council's delays in instituting medical assistance was that all available departmental funds and attention were going to their pet project, a tramway system. [60]

Meanwhile the syndicat was preparing its own system and lobbying with important sources of support. They failed to get the support of local mayors who remained skeptical toward the Landais system; but were more successful with the local branch of the A.G.M.F., *(Association générale des Médecins français)*. The system the syndicat originally planned was the Landais, but by the end of the decade the problems with this system in neighboring departments were well known. The doctors doubted the departmental council would ever adopt it, and therefore proposed an alternative system calling for free choice of doctors and patients and yearly stipends based upon five francs per indigent enlisted, with extra payments for emergency care, bone setting, and surgery. This plan, proposed in 1899, was frustrated by the prefect's refusal to present it to the council, and in July 1901 the syndicat notified the prefect by letter that they would cease treating indigents. To show they meant it the doctors also sent similar written notification to their indigent clients telling them that unless they could produce a letter from their mayor stating that the commune would pay their medical bills they would no longer be cared for free of charge. The prefect responded by calling a special session of the departmental council in March of 1902 in which the council charged a commission with formulating a system. Following the commission's recommendation, the council voted simply to create a budget, turn the whole problem of administration over to the syndicat, and let them organize their own system. [61] The *Union des Syndicats médicaux de France* heralded this as

a

"great syndicat victory, the first time a doctors' syndicat has received an official investiture...Let us hope that the socialization of medicine which we must submit to sooner or later, because it makes more progress every day, will cause health functions to fall to medical syndicats, rather than causing medicine to fall to *fontionnarisme.* [62]

Thus the Union clearly saw the control of local doctors over their department's medical assistance systems as a barrier to socialized medicine. The success of the doctors' syndicat of Lot-et-Garonne far exceeded their own expectations.

Another strike movement promoted by *La Fédération médicale* took place in Tarn whose syndicat joined the federation in 1896 at the urging of the Haute-Garonne syndicat. In 1896 the Tarn syndicat asked for a change in the department Landais system so that doctors would receive additional fees for surgery, increased travel fees and fees for childbirth as well as the abolition of mayors' controls over prescriptions. These demands backfired as the prefect played upon the general hostility of the council toward doctors to have himself granted full powers in organizing the medical assistance system. He appointed a commission to study the issue, and following his own wishes, the commission abolished the Landais system. To replace it they created a circumscription system which paid yearly stipends to doctors computed on the basis of the number of indigents enlisted in the doctor's area. The doctors would receive 1.50 francs per enlisted indigent living within two kilometers of his home, two francs for those living five to ten kilometers away, and 3.50 francs for those living more than ten kilometers away.

There would be also a ten franc subsidy for surgery. [63]

The Tarn syndicat was particularly angered by the fact that three doctor-councilors had supported the prefect's reorganization. Upon the motion of Dr. Jaurès, the syndicat voted to censure these three fellow doctors. [64] In 1897 the syndicat warned the prefect that the new system was "...incompatible with the professional dignity of physicians," and circulated an advisory to all department doctors telling them not to participate in the new program. [65] From the Fall of 1897 to the following August, most Tarn doctors went on strike against the system, although most also continued to treat indigents without charge. Ultimately a new commission, appointed by the departmental council, returned to the Landais system and instituted all the reforms the doctors had requested. Fees for visits outside a one kilometer radius from the doctor's home were raised to two francs; an additional tariff schedule was adopted so that doctors would receive six to twenty francs for childbirth and 10 francs for surgery. The mayors' approval of prescriptions was abolished. [66]

Hérault was not part of *La Fédération médicale* but the departmental medical syndicat belonged to the *Union des Syndicats médicaux de France*. Like their neighboring syndicalist in the federation, however, Hérault doctors had to contend with one of the highest rates of doctors per population in the nation. In 1889 the syndicat first met to draw up a list of demands in anticipation of the Medical Assistance Law. These included free choice of doctors, payment by visit, and suppression of other medical assistance systems which existed in some communes.

The Landais system was subsequently put into effect in some parts of the department but the departmental council and prefect were quickly dismayed by high expenses and began to plan a new system based upon cicumscriptions. The prefect complained that the doctors' bills included charges for surgery, a supplement not provided for under the departmental system. He also charged that doctors were exaggerating their travel expenses by charging for the distance between their homes and the homes of each indigent visited in the same location although they had seen them on the same day. [67] In 1895 the syndicat held a meeting at Montpellier to protest. The doctors complained that under the new system a lot of bogus indigents would be enlisted who were currently paying clients. [68]

In January of 1896 the circumscription system was put into effect in Hérault. Indigents were allowed to choose their doctor; stipends were determined by the number of indigents enlisted for each doctor with adjustments made for the topography of each area. In August 1899 the prefect reported that most midwives and pharmacists had agreed to the system, but that many doctors refused to participate. The result was that of eighty-five medical circumscriptions, thirty-four had no doctors serving medical assistance. The prefect expressed the belief that the doctors did not truly object to the system and would go along if fees were raised. [69] The doctors' non-cooperation continued until 1901, with the syndicat meanwhile discussing a formal strike. In that year, however, they reached an agreement with the departmental council whereby fees were raised from a base of 1.91 francs per enlisted person to 2.83, with the adoption of the Girondin surgical fee schedule. The prefect appeased the doctors' fears of losing paying clients by stipulating that there would be an investigation of lists in any circumscription where enrollments were over 5.75 per cent of the population. Nevertheless in 1902 there were still a number of doctors holding out against the system because of their steadfast allegiance to the Landais system. [70]

Of the fifty-five departments for which information on the functioning of medical assistance at the local level was gathered for this study, seventeen experienced actual strikes or threatened strikes by doctors over medical assistance. This occurred in spite of the fact that Article Fourteen of the 1892 law on the practice of medicine, an amendment made by the Senate, made strikes of the physicians' syndicats against any government authority illegal; however, only one member of the C.S.A.P., Jules de Crisenoy, noted this fact and no syndicat was prosecuted for striking over medical assistance. [71] In addition to the syndicat actions already described in Haute-Loire, Lot-et-Garonne, Ariège, Aveyron, Hautes-Pyrenées and Tarn, similar actions took place in Aube, Calvados, Cantal, Corréze, Eure-et-Loir, Ille-et-Vilaine, Manche, Morbihan, Sarthe, Seine-Inférieure, Seine-et-Marne, and the Vendée. These strikes principally involved efforts to promote the Landais system and, secondly, to raise fees.

In Manche and Cantal doctors successfully blocked plans to switch systems from the Landais system to circumscriptions. In 1894 Cantal adopted payment by stipend but doctors organized and refused to participate, with the result that the Landais system was adopted the following year. Between 1896 and 1899 there were considerable complaints from departmental officials about abuses under the Landais system. They protested specifically that doctors prescribed medicine which was unneccessarily costly and refused to hospitalize chronic cases, but the Landais system remained in effect. [72]

In Seine-Inférieure, where departmental authorities had attempted to institute a dispensary system for rural areas, the communes were very resistant to the Landais system. [73] In 1895, 580 of 700 communes were reported to be applying medical assistance poorly or not at all; 144 other communes spent their full year's budget in six months. In that same year there was a strong contingent in the departmental council that wanted to abolish the Landais system but they were blocked by a commission headed by Emile Ferry. Ferry told the council, "Physicians are a precious ally of the state, as much or more for their moral influence as for their medical influence." [74] The council did authorize the prefect to allow communes with very high medical assistance expenses to change to a stipend system; 172 attempted to do so but doctors responded by refusing to cooperate. [75] A similar situation transpired in Eure-et-Loir, when the departmental council allowed communes to choose between the two systems, but doctors successfully insisted on the Landais system. [76]

In Ille-et-Vilaine the department tried the Landais system in 1895 but switched to the circumscription system the following year after several communes spent three times their allotted budget for medical assistance. In 1899 doctors at Montfort and St. Malo organized a strike against the system which eventually spread to most of the department. They refused to accept an offer by the prefect to raise their yearly stipends from .85 francs per inscribed indigent to one franc. The council responded by creating a new system which allowed for free choice of doctors and indigents while maintaining stipends and circumscriptions. Doctors accepted this system since free choice was a crucial issue to the doctors as 11.24 per cent of the population was enrolled as eligible under medical assistance. Under this revised system the doctor was able to refuse service to indigents they felt should not be eligible. [77]

In the department of Aube the council adopted a circumscription system in 1896. Syndicat doctors accepted it provisionally, providing that the Landais system be adopted the following year. Dr. Bordes of the council urged the Landais system, warning his colleagues that the adoption of the circumscription system "amounted to a declaration of war between doctors and the administration." He claimed he was "... the flag bearer of a plethora of young doctors who are prepared to resist...they will show you that medical solidarity is not in vain. We will make your system impossible." [78] Apparently the doctors lived up to Bordes' words for by 1899 only fifty-five per cent of Aube's population (two-thirds of the communes) were participating in medical assistance and of the participating population only 2.78 per cent was enlisted as eligible. In 1899 the council tried to settle the issue by leaving it up to the communes to make separate arrangements with doctors. [79]

In Morbihan and Sarthe syndicat strike efforts failed to get the Landais system substituted for circumscription systems. In Sarthe, doctors were concerned over the connection made in that department between the service to protect infants and medical assistance. Both services had been in effect since 1855, but medical assistance was enacted by merely extending medical services to the families of children enlisted under the other services. Doctors demanded both the Landais system and the separation of the two services but failed in the face of extreme hostility against them in the departmental council. [80]

In Morbihan doctors struggled for nearly ten years with the departmental council over medical assistance. In 1894 the council adopted a circumscription system which the syndicat rejected. A conciliation commission failed to reach an agreement acceptable to both. Doctors insisted on the Landais system but the council felt the low number of practitioners in the department made it infeasible (one practitioner per 7039, which was third to lowest rate in the nation). Several communes were fifteen to twenty-eight kilometers away from the nearest doctor. The council offered what they considered generous stipends of 1,200 to 2,000 francs but doctors vowed that they would not be the only department in Brittany without the Landais system. [81]

In 1898 Morbihan adopted a "systeme kilometrique" which the syndicat accepted whereby doctors were paid a stipend and travel supplement based upon the distance from their residence to the indigents they visited. However, this system was made optional to the communes, and when 29 of 254 communes refused to adopt it, the doctors refused to service those communes. The council felt that doctors should serve all communes regardless of their choice of system, telling doctors in effect that they could not "...impose their will on the communes." [82] Between 1898-1901 medical assistance apparently did function in part of the department, although no statistics were reported to the Ministry of Interior. In 1901 the syndicat finally voted to go along with the 1898 system. [83]

In Cavados, Seine-et-Marne and the Vaucluse, where the Landais system was promptly adopted, doctors threatened strikes over fees. In 1895 in Calvados, the council's medical assistance fee schedule was accepted by only twenty-five of the department's 147 doctors. The council was forced to increase the supplementary payments for surgery (from five to fifty francs) and for fractures (from twenty to fifty francs). [84] In 1895 as well, Seine-et-Marne doctors settled for an increase of fees from one to two francs for night visits and 1.50 francs supplements for minor surgery. [85] In the Vendée three-quarters of the department's doctors organized against the department's decision to make proportional reductions of all doctor's bills which went over the amount budgeted. Doctors demanded and got a twenty per cent maximum set upon the amount of reductions which could be made. [86] The doctors' concern over fees indicates that medical assistance programs could make an important impact on their economic situations.

Among all departments, between 1895 and 1899, doctors' fees under the Landais system were typically one franc to 1.50 francs for visits during the day and two to three francs for visits at night. Usually travel was also reimbursed at 0.50 francs to one franc per kilometer for trips over one or two kilometers distance from the doctor's residence. [87] These fees only were paid for visits to the homes of the indigent patients. Under most Landais systems doctors were supposed to set aside certain hours during the week or month in which they would see indigents free of charge. The usual fees for rural doctors in the south for peasants and workers were about three francs per visit. [88] Thus medical assistance fees in combination with travel supplements were not far below the doctors' regular fees.

Under circumscription and cantonal systems stipends were generally based upon the number of indigents inscribed and usually ranged from two to three francs per eligible indigent although some departments initially paid only one to 1.50 francs. In addition, some departments with these systems also paid travel at 0.50 to one franc per kilometer beyond a reasonable distance (usually 2 kilometers.) [89]

It is difficult to arrive at a clear picture of what doctors under these systems actually received per year because of the lack of information on how many doctors in a department participated under cantonal and circumscription systems, and how many patients they had on their lists. In the city of Rhône, doctors working under the home care program of the *Bureau de Bienfaisance* received a stipend of 2000 francs a year. [90] In Alpes-Maritimes in 1885-1889 cantonal doctors received 1,000 to 3,000 francs per year. [91] In Eure-et-Loir under the pre-1893 dispensary system, the doctor of one canton received 400 francs a year while that of a second received 800 and a third canton paid their doctor 1,200. In 1894

Haute-Garonne doctors received from 300 to 1,200 francs a year; in Meurthe-et-Moselle, 650 to 775; in Hautes-Alpes 100 to 700 plus travel expenses of one franc per kilometer. [92]   According to the medical press of the time, most rural doctors earned between 2,000 to 2,500 francs a year so the monies to be made from medical assistance were a significant addition to their income. [93] *Le Concours* claimed that 4,000 francs was the minimum salary that rural doctors should make in order to be able to maintain the proper life style so these added funds must have been very welcome. [94]

In many departments there were strong complaints over expenses incurred by medical assistance programs. In twenty-two of the fifty-five departments in the sample, officials complained of abuses of the system and overly high fees charged by doctors and pharmacists. In 20 (ninety-five per cent) of these twenty-two departments a Landais system, or modified version of the Landais system, was in effect. [95] (Overall fifty-seven per cent of the departments used the Landais system in 1899.) [96] Thus the Landais system, favored by doctors, was the most likely to cause financial abuses.

Most complaints involved accusations of too many visits and over-prescribing. Several observers noted that competition of doctors for patients resulted in too many prescriptions being written because patients expected to be given medicines and favored the doctors who prescribed the most. The Landais system and mixed systems, in which doctors were chosen by the patients, were particularly liable to this abuse. [97] In 1898, in one commune in the department of Lot, five patients cost a total of 721 francs in doctor's fees and pharmacy bills. In another commune in the same department, where the inhabitants numbered about 1200, the total pharmacy bill for medical assistance came to 985 francs. [98] In Cantal twenty per cent of treated indigents were found to have cost the system an average of one hundred francs each in three to four months' time. [99] In some cases it was clear that the doctor's patients were involved in fraud with at least the tacit knowledge of their practitioner. In Aude an inspector paid a surprise visit to the home of one indigent patient who was turning in prescriptions for large amounts of cod liver oil to discover that the patient was lighting his home with it. [100] In other cases it was clear that patients were engaging in selling the substances they were being prescribed. [101] The inspector in Lot complained that one person was given prescriptions for "...enough opium to put ten Chinese to sleep." [102] In Cantal one indigent patient used up seven kilograms of hydrophillic cotton in fifteen days, worth seventy francs. Another patient with an "ordinary illness" cost eight francs in doctor's fees and 340 francs in pharmacy fees in four months. His pharmacy bill included ninety francs for opium. [103] In one commune in Puy-de-Dôme a doctor prescribed one kilogram of chocolate for each indigent on his list. [104] The departmental inspector for public assistance claimed there was a black market in drugs and food paid for by medical assistance resulting from a conspiracy between pharmacists, doctors and indigents. [105]

Apparently some indigents were using their doctor's willingness to prescribe to supply their families with mineral water and table wine free of charge. In Cantal an inspector reported that wine and mineral water was being prescribed five to ten bottles per prescription, along with "exotic and tasty syrups". [106] Similar cases were reported in several other departments. [107] In Dordogne and Pas-de-Calais, inspectors reported several cases of conspiracy and kickbacks between doctors and pharmacists. [108] Fees for travel expenses created problems because of abuses whereby doctors would charge for the distance from their home or office to each indigent visited in the same village or hamlet even though they had visited them all in the same trip. [109]

The Union and *Le Concours* objected strongly to complaints that doctors were making too many visits under the Landais system. Reporting to the annual assembly of the Union of syndicats in 1903, Dr. René Millon observed that such complaints were due to the prejudices "of the bougeoisie, ... of the philosophes ... against the doctors of the countryside." [110] He blamed the prejudices of the elite doctors in each department who were inspectors of medical assistance, and were also usually on the departmental councils and control commission for medical assistance. Millon mentioned in particular the situations in Ille-et-Vilaine and the Vaucluse where he claimed elite doctors were persecuting their more lowly brothers who participated in medical assistance systems. He also criticized Monod for the latter's comments in the C.S.A.P. 1899 report on medical assistance where he said some doctors were making too many visits. If a few doctors were visiting some indigents too often, Millou argued, it was only because they were trying to recoup income lost by treating indigents who the mayors refused to make eligible for assistance. [111]

Doctors and pharmacists were not always responsible for abuses of the system. In Aisne the prefect reported a fraud engaged in by a mayor of a commune. The mayor was enlisting families as eligible for assistance who were well able to pay for their medical care, and then collecting kickbacks from the families. [112]

Gradually departments began to control expenses by appointing inspectors and control committees to investigate high bills. In Dordogne in 1899, Dr. Jammés was appointed *Médecin controller* of the medical assistance program. His report documents prevalent problems in carrying out medical assistance. Dordogne had a Landais system, controlled by the mayors by a system of chits. Jammés found the mayors to be very lax in performing the required paperwork for the chits and doctors and mayors alike were very uncooperative in writing the diagnosis and prognosis of their indigent patients as the chits required. Jammés found doctors also generally refused to report their planned course of treatment, also as required. [113]

Jammés found extensive lack of compliance in the department; sixty-five communes made no lists. Overall the number of indigents enlisted for treatment was lower than that expected by the departmental council and the cost was higher. Dr. Jammés attributed this to doctors making too many visits and over-prescribing, which he blamed on the greed of doctors practicing in the same area who "competed to turn in the highest bills." [114] In one commune, Jammés found a fraud which had been carried by a pharmacist and doctor in collusion. Alarmed by the high number of illness reports and pharmacy bills, Jammés visited some of the supposed patients only to discover they had never been ill and never seen the doctor. He also discovered several other petty frauds on the part of pharmacists, such as altering the doctors' prescriptions to increase the amounts and substituting a more expensive medicine, such as fancy mineral water for the local supply. There were also some cases of pharmacists forging prescriptions. Jammés' inspection reduced pharmacists' and doctors' bills by ten per cent. He pointed out that in spite of this the program was still over budget and was only continuing to function on surpluses from the hospital budget. [115]

The inspectors and control commissions took a variety of measures in order to deal with what was seen as the excessive costs of medical assistance programs. Several departments amended their programs so that abusive doctors and pharmacists could be excluded from participating. [116] They cautioned doctors to hospitalize patients with chronic or long-term illnesses which would otherwise require many visits and high pharmacy expenses. [117] The Union, however, continued to take a strong position against hospitalization of indigents under medical assistance programs. In 1901 the Union warned doctors that hospitals, "contrary to the spirit of the law," were treating far too many medical assistance patients. They took the position that minor surgery on indigents should be performed by the home care physician in the indigent's home. The Union also demanded that hospital physicians respect the "rights" of the private doctor who first started an indigent patient's treatment, once that patient returned home from the hospital. [118] In spite of the fears of the Union and the efforts of the inspectors and control commissions to encourage utilization of hospitals, the number of indigents hospitalizaed under the medical assistance programs was quite small. The percentage of indigents hospitalized measured as a per cent of the total indigents treated ranged from 0.2 to 5.9 per cent but averaged 2.0 per cent. [119] There was no significant difference in the average percentage of indigents hospitalized between the circumscription and Landais systems. However, it is interesting to note that the departments where the syndicats were affiliated with *La Fédération médicale* had significantly lower rates of hospitalization than the rest of the nation, with an average of 1.4 per cent of indigents treated being hospitalized. [120] This finding suggests that in areas of intense competition for clients, doctors were less likely to send their patients to hospitals and thus lose their patronage to hospital doctors.

The departments usually required doctors not to take primary responsibility for childbirth but rather to leave this to midwives. Under most systems doctors were only to be called in cases of difficult births, or in the absence of any licensed midwives. In a few departments it was left up to the midwife to make the decision to call a doctor. [121] The Union of syndicats objected to this regulation because "the pushing off of pregnant women on midwives is not fair to the patient." [122] The emphasis on payment for services rendered and free choice was not generally extended to midwives who often continued to operate under circumscription and cantonal systems while the doctors operated under the Landais system. [123] Midwives did not gain from the medical assistance system to nearly the same extent as doctors and pharmacists; payments to midwives amounted to about 3.0 per cent of the total budgets for home care under medical assistance programs in 1899, as compared to 49.0 per cent for doctors and 48.0 per cent for pharmacists. [124]

The major way of dealing with problems of high expenses was by making proportional reductions in the reimbursements to doctors and pharmacists when the total bills went over the medical assistance budget. In some departments these reductions amounted to twenty to fifty per cent of the doctors' fees. [125] Between 1896 and 1897 reductions affected forty-eight per cent of doctors in Charente-Inférieure, thirty-one per cent in Loire-Inférieure and forty-five per cent in Lot. [126]

In 1899 seventy-six per cent of the departments with Landais systems made proportional reductions on the bills of their doctors and parmacists. Of departments with cantonal systems, only thirty-three per cent were forced to make such reductions. [127] Even after these reductions were made, the Landais system was more expensive to operate than the cantonal. The average cost of home care treatment per each indigent cared for under the Landais systems was 16.30 francs as compared with a cost of 13.80 under the cantonal systems, a statistically significant difference (see Table V-1). [128] This difference coincides with the pattern established for the two systems before 1893. [129] Further, as was also true of the two systems before 1893, the cantonal systems were more effective in reaching indigents than the Landais systems. In 1899 under the cantonal systems an average of 6.4 per cent of the participating populations were enlisted as eligible for medical assistance, a figure quite close to the C.S.A.P. estimate of the actual per cent of the French population in need of assistance (6.2 per cent). Under the Landais system however the average was only 3.9 per cent. Again, the difference is significant (see Table V-1). [130]

By the end of the century there were some new trends in the administration of medical assistance. In a few departments between 1895 and 1900 the administration abolished the Landais system in favor of circumscription systems. [131] However the strongest trend was for departments to abandon the idea of a department-wide system and leave it up to the communes to make arrangements with their local practitioners on how the system would operate. This occurred in about thirty-two per cent of the departments by 1900. [132] Even in those departments which maintained departmental systems, communes could take advantage of article thirty-five of the 1893 law which provided for dispensation from its requirements if a commune could prove it had an adequate system of its own for assuring medical assistance. By 1899 the C.S.A.P. was faced with an increasing number of requests from communes for exemptions under this article. [133]

The doctors' syndicats were overwhelmingly successful in promoting their interests at the national level but at the local level they met serious resistance. In the period 1888-1902 the syndicat movement of doctors spread to virtually every department, and doctors generally displayed a close unity of aims and interests. The themes of free choice, payment by visit, the abolition of *médecins-fonctionnaires,* were raised by the Union and *Le Concours* and were echoed everywhere by local syndicats. In contrast to this unity of doctors, local communities in France displayed wide dissimilarities in attitudes toward doctors and towards modern medicine and state assistance programs. Furthermore, between the level of departmental and national government there was a clear dichotomy between the views of the majority of national legislators and many departmental councillors. At the national level it was assumed that the medical and social contact of doctors and rural people was an end to be greatly desired. At the local level this was seriously questioned.

In spite of this resistance, physicians' syndicats were remarkably successful in promoting their view of medical assistance. The Landais system became the dominant form of application of the law even though in 1899 as in 1887 the Landais system was clearly more costly and less efficient than the cantonal system. It is perhaps a measure of the doctors' growing political influence at the departmental level, that generally departments were not able overtly to abolish the Landais system but rather chose to simply allow communes to evade it if they could.

The medical assistance issue was a major impetus to the professional organization of physicians at the local level. These local syndicats were not temporary but rather a permanent lobbying base which latter extended their activity to other issues. [134] Thus, in this period physicians' syndicats became a powerful medical and political force at the national and local level. They used this power to promote the Landais system of medical assistance and thus to use the government to expand liberal private practice at the expense of traditional collective forms of care.

Table V-I

Functioning of Medical Assistance Under
Different Systems in 1899*

System	Number of Departments	Indigents Eligible: Average Percent of Total Population	Indigents Treated: Average Percent of Indigents Eligible	Average Expenses per Indigent Treated
Landais	46	3.9%	33.3%	16.2 francs
Cantonal	13	6.4%	36.9%	13.8 francs
Mixed	23	5.4%	37.3%	17.0 francs
All	82	4.7%	35.0%	16.0 francs

*Conseil supérieur d'Assistance publique, Fascicule 92, Tableaux I,II. Archives de la Santé publique, Paris. Corse was left out of this study (see notes to Table 2).

Note: The Mann-Whitney test (see notes to Table 2), revealed that the difference in the means between the Landais and Cantonal systems for Indigents Eligible, Indigents Treated, and Expenses per Indigent Treated was significant.

NOTES TO CHAPTER V

1. After 1893 the term "Vosgian system" was more commonly used to refer to the Landais system, that is, the system which included free choice of practitioner and payment by visit. The term Landais was discredited ultimately because of the fact that the department of Landes had abandonned the system. I have continued to use the term Landais system to describe developments between 1893 and 1902 for the sake of clarity.

2. Conseil supérieur de l'Assistance publique, Fasiscule 9, n.d., "Médecine gratuite en faveur des indigents des campagnes, tableau 2, fonctionnement en 1887, (hereinafter, C.S.A.P., Fasc. 9); C.S.A.P., Fasc. 92, "Rapport sur l'Assistance médicale gratuite pendant les années 1897, 1898, and 1899, Tableau III, 1899, pp 54-57, 35-37; the Statistics utilized in this chapter for the pre-1893 systems refers to the thirty-seven departments for which information on medical assistance in 1887 is available from the records of the C.S.A.P. (fasc 9, see above). In 1887 five departments had the Landais system, twenty-four the cantonal system and eight had mixed systems. The statistics for the post 1893 systems is drawn from 81 departments for which information on medical assistance in 1899 is available. At this time forty-six

departments used the Landais system, thirteen the cantonal system, and twenty-two had mixed systems.

3. The circumscription system which came into use after 1893, was a modification of the old cantonal system. The departments started using various groupings of communes rather than the traditional cantons to form areas for medical assistance jurisdictions. In essence the systems were quite similar, one or two doctors were appointed to serve the indigents of a particular area and the doctors were paid according to a yearly stipend.

4. de Crisenoy, *Questions,* 1898 pp 129-130 Similar difficulties were reported in Lozére, Morbihan and Loire.

5. Lessieur; C.S.A.P., Fasc. 92. The density of practitioners in the city of Brioude comes to 1/2142 if the surburban cantons are included); the density in Le Puy equals 1/3630 if the suburban cantons are included.

6. de Crisenoy, *Questions* 1898 p 199; 1895 p 200; 1899 p 84; C.S.A.P. Fasc. 92, p 18.

7. de Crisenoy, *Questions* 1895 p 182.

8. *Ibid.* 1896 pp 152-53; 1888 156-58.

9. *La France médicale,* V. 39, N. 39 (Sept. 23, 1892) p 621; *Le Concours,* V. 14, N. 4 (Jan 23, 1892) pp 47-48; V. 14 N. 45 (Nov. 5, 1892) pp 53-54; de Crisenoy, *Questions,* 1895 n.p.

10. The other co-founder was Dr. Le Baron. Auguste de Cézilly was also closely associated with the founding of the Union: "Nécrologie: M. le Dr. Fourmestreaux, *Bul. Off. de l'Union des Syn. méd. de Fr.,* N.

11, (June 5, 1902), pp 201-02.

11. *Ibid.;* A highly urbanized department, Seine-et-Oise had several cities with active *bureaux de bienfaisance* with more or less effective medical assistance programs attached. These communes were therefore exempted from the department's program of medical assistance.

12. Dr. Giberton, "Syndicat médical de l'Arrondissement de Versailles," *Bulletin des Syndicats,* (May 1899) pp 769-772.

13. C.S.A.P., Fasc. 92.

14. de Crisenoy, *Questions* 1888 pp 350-351; 1889 203-205; Dr. Giberton, "Syndicat médical de l'Arrondissement de Versailles," *Bulletin des Syndicats,* (May 1899) pp 769-772.

15. 2.12 per cent of the population was enlisted as indigents versus a national average of 4.7 per cent and the C.S.A.P. figure of 6.24 per cent, which was its estimate of true indigency; C.S.A.P., Fasc. 92, p 12.

16. de Crisenoy, *Questions,* 1888 p 161.

17. *Ibid.*

18. Dr. Roland, "Rapport de Dr. Roland," de Crisenoy, *Questions,* 1890, pp 202-204; Dr. Roland also repored that the council had received bills from unlicensed practitioners, so called bandigists, whom they refused to reimburse.

19. Dr. Guillon, "l'Assistance médicale dans la Vienne," *Le Concours,* 13 année, n. 46, (14 Nov. 1891). p 7.

20. de Crisenoy, *Questions* 1892, p 206; 1896, p 172.

21. M. Garin, "Du Service sanitaire de Lyon, sa organisation et ses resultats pratiques," *Lyon médical,* N. 19 (April 31, 1878) pp 37-40; N. 20 (May 19, 1878) pp 86-101; N. 21 (May 26, 1878) pp 120-130; P. Diday, "Assistance médicale devant le Conseil général du Rhône," *Lyon médical* N. 21 (April 31, 1878). The pages of *Lyon médical* in the late 1870s trace a heated controversy over the inspection of prostitutes. The justness of the task was never questioned but the head of the *Service sanitaire,* Dr. Garin, was under heavy attack for his lack of thoroughness in rounding up prostitutes.

22. Dr. Carry, "Histoire du Syndicat de l'Association des Médecins du Rhône," *Bulletin official de Syndicat des Médecins du Rhône,* (Oct. 1902) pp 185-86.

23. Crisenoy, *Questions,* 1895 p 213.

24. P. Diday, "Assistance médicale devant le Conseil général du Rhône," *Lyon médical* (August 31, 1878) p 71. Several other councilors also expressed the view that if medical assistance was enacted its funds should be used to pay unlicensed practitioners as well; *Ibid.* pp 72-72.

25. Dr. Carry, "Histoire du Syndicat de l'Association des Médecins du Rhône," *Bulletin Official de Syndicat des Médecins du Rhône,* (Oct. 1902) p 185-186; The syndicat had been urging the department council for several years to take action in advance of the laws going into effect, however the council delayed, in part, because of an on going battle between it and the *Hôtel Dieu* of Lyon. The *Hôtel Dieu* had lately been designated as a departmental hospital, requiring, therefore, that it admit

all indigents in the department free of charge. The hospital was fighting to revert to its original designation as a communal hospital because the 1893 law required communes without hospitals designated for them to budget money for the care of their indigents at the nearest hospital. Under the designation as departmental hospital, the *Hôtel Dieu* of Rhône was not eligible for these funds. The council finally voted to table this issue until medical assistance was organized "Bulletin, Rapport de commission de Conseil général, Loi 15 Juillet 1893," *Lyon médical,* N. 36 (Sept. 6, 1896) pp 23-33.

26. "Variétés: Assistance médicale gratuite," *Lyon Médical* N. 1 (Jan 5, 1896) pp 33-34.

27. "Bulletin" *Lyon médical* N. 1 (Jan 5, 1896) pp 26-33; Dr. Carrey, "Histoire du Syndicat de l'Association des Médecins du Rhône," *Bulletin official du syndicat des Médecins du Rhône,* (OCt. 1902) p 185-86.

28. de Crisenoy, *Questions,* 1898 130-133.

29. "Assemblée des médecins de l'Arrondissement de Villefranche-sur-Saône," (A subdivision of the Syndicat des médecins du Rhône), Dec. 2, 1900, *Bulletin des Syndicats médicaux de France et des Sociétés locales,* (Fev. 1901) pp 1022-1023.

30. "Variétés, l'Assistance médicale gratuite," *Lyon médical,* N. 45 (Nov. 8, 1896). n.p.

31. Dr. Carry, *Ibid.*

32. Dr. Carrey, *Ibid.;* "Intérêts professionnels," *Le Provence médical* (June 14, 1902).

33. de Crisenoy, *Questions,* 1889, p 192-93; 1893, n.p.

34. *Ibid.,* 1896 pp 161-164.

35. *Bulletin des Sociétés médicales de France et* des Sociétés locales, (Sept. 1899) pp 817-819.

36. de Crisenoy, *Questions,* 1895 p 218.

37. "Assistance médicale gratuite en Mayenne," *Rev. des Et. de Bien.,* July 1897 p 187; "l'Assistance médicale gratuite en Lot-et-Garonne," *Rev. des Et. de Bien.,* Oct. 1899, p 326; C.S.A.P., Fasc. 92, p 11.

38. Eure, Tarn, Vienne, Lot-et-Garonne, Mayenne: de Crisenoy, *Questions,* 1896 p 172.

39. de Crisenoy, *Questions,* pp 178-79.

40. *Ibid.,* 1893 p 195.

41. *Ibid.,* pp 152-175.

42. Millon, op. cit.

43. de Crisenoy, *Questions* p 172-173.

44. *Ibid.*

45. *Ibid., 1898 p 113; C.S.A.P., Fasc. 92.*

46. Dr. Clavelier, "La Fédération des syndicats médicaux du Sud-Ouest," *La Fédération mdicale,* (hereinafter, *La Féd. méd.* N. 56 (Mars 1901), n.p.; N. 54, (Jan 1901); N. 18 (Jan. 1898); C.S.A.P., Fasc. 92.

47. Dr. Lucien Dore, "l'Assistance médicale dans la Haute-Garonne," *La Féd. méd.,* N. 5, (Oct. 1897) pp 3-6.

48. Dr. Lucien Dore, *La Féd. méd.*, N. 6, (Jan 1897) pp 1-2; N. 9 (April 1897) pp 5-9; N. 58 (May 1901) pp 3-4; De Crisenoy, *Questions* 1896 p 158.

49. Dr. Scalp, "Le Conseil d'Assistance," *La Féd. méd.* N. 12, (July 1897), n.p.

50. "Association des syndicats des Médecins de la Haute-Garonne," *Bul. des syn Méd de France,* (Sept. 1899) pp 819-821; "Syndicat de Lot-et-Garonne," *Bul. Off. de l'Union,* N. 21, (Nov. 1903), p 423.

51. *La Féd. méd., N. 58, (May 1901) pp 3-7.*

52. *de Crisenoy, 1899,* pp 88-91.

53. "Lutte contre le Conseil général de l'Ariège au sujet de l'organisation du service d'assistance médicale," *Bul. des Syn. méd. de Fr.,* p 879; Dec 1900, p 797; May 1900 pp 913-914;

54. *La Féd. méd.* N. 19 (Feb. 1898).

55. *Ibid.; Bulletin des Syn. méd. de Fr.,* August 1899, p 807; de Crisenoy, *Questions,* 1895 pp 176-77.

56. Crisenoy, 1895, p 212; *La Féd. méd* N. 14 (Sept 1897).

57. *La Féd méd,* N. 28 (Nov. 1898) pp 11-13.

58. C.S.A.P., Fasc. 92, p 11.

59. C.S.A.P., Fasc. 92 p 10.

60. de Crisenoy, 1898, pp 122-123; "Assistance médicale-gratuite, Lot-et-Garonne," *Rev. des Et. de Bien.,* (Oct. 1899) p 326; "Syndicat médical de Lot-et-Garonne" *Bul. des Syn méd de Fr.* (July 1901) pp

1081-1082.

61. "Syndicat Médical de Lot-et-Garonne, Assistance médicale gratuite,: *Bul. des Syn. Méd. de Fr.* (April 1899) pp 756-58; (July 1901) pp 1081-82; "Syndicat médical de Lot-et-Garonne," *La Féd. méd,* N. 61 (Aug. 1901) p 3; N. 64 (Nov. 1901) pp 8-11; N. 72 (July 1902) pp 10-11.

62. "Syndicat de Lot-et-Garonne," *Bul. Off. de l'Union,* N. 21, (Nov. 1903), p 423.

63. "Commission de l'Assistance médicale gratuite, Réunion de 29 Oct. 1898," *La Féd. méd.,* N. 228, (Nov. 1898), pp 9-10.

64. Dr. Bonneville, "Syndicat du Tarn," *La Féd. méd.,* N. 4, (Sept. 1897) pp 10-12; N. 13, (August 1897).

65. *Ibid.*

66. "l'Assistance médicale dans le Tarn," *La Féd. méd.,* N. 13, (August 1897), pp 6-13; N. 25 (August 1898); de Crisenoy, *Questions* 1899 pp 134.

67. C.S.A.P., Fasc. 92, pp 225.

68. *Bul. des Syn. méd. de Fr.* N. 33 (1889) p 271; de Crisenoy, *Questions,* 1895 p 196-7.

69. Crisenoy, *Questions,* 1899, pp 108-110; *Bul. off. des Syn. méd. de France* (Jan 8, 1901), p 1024; N. 7 (April 1902) pp 128-129.

70. *Ibid.*

71. de Crisenoy, *Questions,* 1896, p 350.

72. *Ibid.,* 1895, p 182; 1896, p 167; 1899 p 95; C.S.A.P., Fasc. 92, p 223.

73. See Chapter III

74. de Crisenoy, *Questions,* 1895 pp 216-218.

75. *Ibid.;* 1898 n.p.; C.S.A.P., Fasc. 92 p 229.

76. de Crisenoy, *Questions* 1895 p 190.

77. *Ibid.,* 1896, p 165, 1899 pp 110-112; C.S.A.P., Fasc. 92 pp 17, 41-42.

78. *Ibid.,* 1895 pp 173-175.

79. C.S.A.P., Fasc. 92 p 18.

80. Dr. Salomon (de Savigne-l'Evêque, Sarthe), "Rapport à la Congrès d'Assistance familiale le sur l'Assistance médicale en famille," *Bul. Off. de l'Union des Syn. méd. de Fr.* (Jan 20, 1902) pp 45-46; de Crisenoy, *Questions,* 1895 pp 214-215.

81. de Crisenoy, *Questions* p 206-208.

82. Ibid., 1898 p 126.

83. C.S.A.P., Fasc. 92 tableau. C.S.A.P., Fasc. 92 p 11.

84. de Crisenoy, *Questions* 1895 pp 177-181.

85. *Ibid.,* pp 218-219;

86. *Ibid.,* 1895 pp 219-220.

87. *La Féd. méd.,* N. 17, (June 1897); N. 13 (Aug. 1897); N. 14 (Sept 1897); *Le Concours,* V. 14 N. 4 (Jan 23, 1892) pp 47-48; V. 14 N. 45

(Nov. 5, 1892) p 53-54; *Bul. Off. des Syn. des Médecins du Rhône* (Oct 1902) pp 180-185; de Crisenoy, *Questions,* 1890 pp 179, 192-196; 1895 p 182, 205; 1898, pp 130-131.

88. de Crisenoy, *Questions,* 1895 pp 173-174.

89. *Ibid.,* 1889, p 136; 1888 pp 193-194; 1889 p 205; 1890 pp 184-185; 1890 pp 180-181; 1895 pp 189-190, 196, 202, 212; 1898 n.p.; 1899 p 10-11; *La Féd. méd.* N. 9 (April 1897) pp 5-8; N. 15 (Oct. 1897) pp 3-4; *Bul. des Syn. méd. de Fr.* (Jan 8, 1901) p 1024.

90. Dr. Carry, "Histoire de syndicat de l'Association des Médecins du Rhône," *Bul. Off. des syn. des Médecins du Rhône,* (Oct 1902) p 185.

91. de Crisenoy, *Questions* 1889 1888-189.

92. *Ibid.,* p 201; 1894 p 183.

93. *Le Courrier médical,* V. 14 N. 11 (March 14, 1891) p 101; *Le Concours,* V. 9, N. 25 (June 18, 1887), pp 293-94.

94. *Le Concours,* op. cit.

95. Landais system: Charente-Inférieure, Côtes-du-Nord, Finistére, Allier, Ardennes, Cantal, Lozére, Maine-et-Loire, Puy-de-Dôme, Seine-Inférieure, Seine-et-Marne, Yonne, Haute-Vienne, Dordogne, Ille-et-Vilaine (switched from Landais to circumscriptions in 1899); Doctors appointed but paid by the visit: Aude, Loire, Rhône; Free choice of doctors but payment by stipend: Lot; Free choice of doctors but payment by a combination of stipend and travel expenses: Hérault; Mixed system (Some communes had Landais, others circumscriptions with a variety of payment methods): Nord; Cantonal: Pas-de-Calais.

96. see p 1 of this chapter.

97. de Crisenoy, *Questions* 1898 pp 120-121; C.S.A.P., Fasc. 92, p 224.

98. de Crisenoy, *Questions* 1898 pp 120-121; C.S.A.P., Fasc. 92, p 227.

99. C.S.A.P., Fasc. 92 p 223.

100. *Ibid.,* 92 p 222.

101. de Crisenoy, *Questions* 1899 p 113, C.S.A.P., Fasc. 92 p 223.

102. *Ibid.,* 1898 pp 120-121.

103. *Ibid.,* 1899 p 95.

104. C.S.A.P., Fasc. 92 p 227.

105. *Ibid.,* 92 p 227.

106. *Ibid., 92 p 223.*

107. *Ibid.,* 92 pp 223-227.

108. de Crisenoy, *Questions* 1891 pp 130-131; 1887 p 135.

109. *Ibid.,* 1898 pp 130-131; C.S.A.P., Fasc. 92 pp 225; for additional information on abuses see: de Crisenoy, 1890 pp 174-175; 1895, p 220 1896, pp 152-153; 1898 pp 135; 1899 p 87-99; C.S.A.P., Fasc. 92, pp 229; "Syndicat des Médecins des Côtes-du-Nord, "Assistance médicale gratuite," *Bul. des Syn. méd. de Fr.* (August 1899) pp 809-811.

110. Dr. René Millon, "Rapport sur le fonctionnement de l'Assistance medicale gratuite dans les départements," *Bul. off. de l'Union des Syn. méd. de Fr.,* N. 21 (Nov. 5, 1902), p 123; N. 23 (Dec. 5, 1903) pp 478-481.

111. *Ibid.*

112. de Crisenoy, *Questions,* 1899 pp 186-87.

113. C.S.A.P., Fasc. 92, p 224.

114. *Ibid.*

115. de Crisenoy, *Questions,* 1899 pp 99-104; C.S.A.P., Fasc. 92, p 17. de Crisenoy, *Questions* 1891 pp 130-131.

116. C.S.A.P., Fasc. 92 p 230.

117. de Crisenoy, *Questions* 1893 p 195; 1899 p 95.

118. *Bul. des Syn. méd. de Fr.,* (June 1901), p 1082.

119. C.S.A.P., Fasc. 92, Tableau IX, pp 100-115; Seine-et-Oise was excluded from the analysis because of its extensive hospital network coupled with the fact that the medical assistance system was not functioning by 1899 in most of the communes (see above). Corse was excluded because its medical system reflected non-French traditions.

120. A Mann-Whitney test was used to test significance of difference of central tendancy; significance was accepted at the <.05 level. There was no significant difference in the percentage of population inscribed as eligible between the departments in *La Fédération médicale de la Sud-Ouest* and the rest of the nation.

121. de Crisenoy *Questions,* 1890 pp 192-192; 1895, 175, 212, 205; 1899 pp 97-98.

122. Dr. Salomon (Savigne-l'Evêque, Sarthe) "Rapport à le Congrès d'Assistance familiale sur l'Assistance médicale en famille," *Bulletin*

Official de l'Union des Syndicats médicaux de France, (Jan 20, 1902).

123. de Crisenoy, *Questions, Ibid.*

124. C.S.A.P., Fasc. 92 Tableau

125. C.S.A.P., Fasc. 92 Tableau

126. Dr. René Millon, "Rapport sur l'Assistance médicale gratuite," *Bul. Off. de l'Union des Syn. méd. de Fr. N. 21,* (Nov. 5, 1902) pp 123-130; N. 22 (Nov. 10, 1902) pp 423-432.

127. This per cent is drawn from the 32 of 42 departments for which this information is available.

128. C.S.A.P., Fasc. 92; See footnote 120 above.

129. See Chapter III.

130. C.S.A.P., Fasc. 92, Tableaux; See footnote 120 above.

131. Five out of the fifty-five departments for which information is available; C.S.A.P., Fasc. 92 pp 17-32; *La Féd. méd.,* N. 28, (Nov. 1898) pp 9-10; de Crisenoy, *Questions,* 1896 p 109.

132. Based upon seventeen of fifty-five departments: C.S.A.P., Fasc. 92 pp 15-40; de Crisenoy, *Questions,* 1896, p 167; 1898, n.p.; Dr. Carrey, "Histoire du Syndicat de l'Association des Medécins du Rhône," *Bulletin officiel des Syndicats des Médecins du Rhône,* Oct. 1902 p 187.

133. C.S.A.P., Fasc. 92.

134. For later issues of syndicat activity see my article: Les Syndicats médicaux et la Mutualité. Le Début du conflit au commencement du vingtième Siècle et l'Exemple du Syndicat Toulousain," *La Revue de l'Economie sociale* (Sept., 1986.).

CONCLUSION

The physicians' Union movement was organized in the late nineteenth century to promote the interests of private practitioners. For several decades these doctors had been looking for ways to redress what they perceived as inadequate social and economic status. The Third Republic presented private practitioners with the opportunity to achieve their professional goals of eliminating competing practitioners, controlling state medicine, and equalizing the profession.

The Union movement reflected the divided nature of the medical profession. The Union movement represented the "médecins du quartier" and the "médecins de campagne" against the "princes of science." * The Union competed with the traditional medical professional organization, the A.G.M.F., and brought up issues which that older organization had refused to address. These issues concerned the social and economic interests of the private practitioners. Under the Union, deontology was construed to address practical issues such as how to manage competition between practitioners to give all doctors a fair

---

* Chapter I, pp 29-31.

chance at clients; the rights of doctors to collect fees and refuse to serve clients who did not pay; the encroachment of specialists and elite doctors into the practice of local doctors; the prosecution of illegal practitioners; and, finally, the protection of the rights of private practice against public health and the *médecins-fonctionnaires*. In essence, the Union worked to increase the monopoly of *docteurs* over medical care and to advance liberal-market medicine on a pay for services rendered basis as the foundation of medical care. The Union succeeded in its goals by carefully harnessing the state to its own ends. State support for collective forms of care were opposed, yet the state was used to expand the doctors' monopoly and to preserve and promote private practice.

As a result of its interaction with the legislature and with the public assistance and public health bureaucracies, the physicians' Union movement of the 1880s and 1890s had a critical impact on the nature of the health care system. The result of this interaction was the hybrid system of private-public medical care. This hybrid structure grew out of the conflict which arose in the late nineteenth century between the professionalization goals of the Union movement and the public health program inspired by the bacteriological revolution. The factor which largely determined the outcome of this conflict was the political ambiance of the Third Republic in this era. Here solidarist-populationist concerns and ideology decided the issue. The solidarists used social reform to oppose the joint threat of socialism and urbanization. The reforms were intended to bring the benefits of scientific progress, as perceived by the governing elites, to all sectors of French society. The desired result was to incorporate all sectors of society into the republican synthesis. Solidarists were of course opposed to any reforms which implied collectivism. They were not in favor of any fundamental change in the social structure, but simply wanted to extend some of the customs and advantages of the middle class to workers and peasants.

Doctors were the natural agents of this program. They held out the promise of scientific progress and yet steadfastly opposed collective relationships. Moreover, private practitioners were the very symbol of the liberal professional and were the trusted political supporters and so often the *élus* of the Third Republic. The medical legislation passed represented the solidarist program to use private practitioners to further the goals of social and political stabilization.

There were many serious social and health problems facing peasants and workers: starvation, malnutrition, poor housing, lack of care for the elderly and handicapped; yet these issues were largely ignored by the legislature. Instead, in 1892 and 1893, the Third Republic passed legislation demanded by the professional-medical lobby which simply increased the monopoly of the private practitioners and expanded their area of practice. Solidarists saw the Medical Practice Law and Medical Assistance Law as a way of bringing supposedly modern medical care to all sectors of the population, especially to rural areas in an effort to stem the flow of population from the countryside into the cities. This reform suited solidarist ideology more than the institution of more basic welfare programs.

For the private-professional Union movement, the medical legislation answered many of the professional problems which had plagued the profession for at least a century. The competition of the *officiers de santé* and illegals would be eliminated; overcrowding in the profession would thus be alleviated; and the doctors would be aided in the collection of fees. The Medical Practice Law gave doctors the monopoly they had long desired and the ability to enforce it. The syndicats were legally recognized and given a special role in identifying and prosecuting illegals. The Union thus became, in effect, a government corporation, as was revealed in Lot-et-Garonne where the local syndicat was given total authority over Medical Assistance. The legal restriction on Union activity which forbade the syndicats to take organized actions against the state, was simply ignored when local syndicats went on strike over medical assistance.

The destruction of the *officiers de santé* was the oldest and probably the most serious goal of the private practitioners. The Union was able to convince Dr. Paul Brouardel and the C.C.H.P. to support this abolition, even though it was recognized that the demise of the *officiers* would have undesirable consequences. In those areas where the *officiers* were still important and numerous, the abolition had a very detrimental impact on the availability of practitioners to the population. Further, the abolition of the *officiers* cut off medical careers to a whole class of society.

Like the Medical Practice Law, the Medical Assistance Law was seen by the physicians' Union as a way of alleviating overcrowding in the profession by expanding the territory in which doctors could make a living. The Medical Assistance Law served other purposes as well, purposes not openly discussed in the legislature, but clearly intended by the Union movement and by many of the members of the C.S.A.P.. Medical Assistance, under the Landais system, would be used to destroy the more collective and traditional cantonal systems, and to block the use of hospitals and dispensaries for indigent care. In planning medical assistance, the C.S.A.P. was dominted by the Union's lobbying in favor of the Landais system in spite of the clear problems with this system. Once the Medical Assistance Law was passed, the Union and bureaucrats cooperated in promoting the Landais system, often against hostile local officials. At the local level, the struggles between doctors' syndicats and officials were often intense and protracted. Using the lines of argument set out by the Union, the local syndicats often succeeded in forcing the Landais system on their departments; however, many of these systems were abused by practitioners and clients and were in serious financial trouble by 1900.

The C.S.A.P. program was in line with the Union movement; the C.C.H.P's was not, and its programs met with much less success. The C.C.H.P. had considerable prestige and important political connections; in the late nineteenth century it found an unprecedented opportunity to put public health measures into effect. The bacteriological revolution was attracting great public attention all over Europe; the discoveries of Pasteur and Koch held out the promise that at last effective measures would be found to stop the devastating course of contagious disease.

The French government was highly motivated to put these measures into effect. Typhoid and cholera were ravaging a nation where the society and culture were already perceived to be fragile and in danger of extinction. Liberal-interventionist ideology of the late nineteenth century supported state involvement in stopping the course of disease and lowering mortality. Solidarists like Henri Monod and Léon Bourgeois carefully explained that in the area of health the welfare of society should outweigh the individual's rights. For their part, the public, or at least the workers and peasants, welcomed state intervention in the form of disinfection services and epidemic services. Private practitioners, however, did not welcome state intervention and seemed to equate society's good health with the expansion of their monopoly over health care.

The program to initiate bacteriological public health was fraught with obstacles. Initially there were scientific and technical problems. The C.C.H.P. had to examine and explain how bacteria were transmitted and to clear the murky waters of confusion between miasma and bacteria. Some of these problems proved surmountable, others did not. However, these were not ultimately the major issues for the legislature. The rights of private property as interpreted by the senate and doctors took precedence over many public health concerns. Previous attempts of the public bureaucaracy, operating under miasma theory, had run into the opposition of property owners and landlords. Bacteriological public health offered a way around such difficulties. Simply by providing cleaner water and better sewage disposal, a great impact could be made on some of the worst diseases. These measures could be carried out by the government with little or no interference in the right of property owners. It was not surprising, therefore, that pure water and vaccination were the only important provisions which were enacted by the Public Health Law of 1902. By the late nineteenth century, it was well recognized that crowded, dark and damp housing also contributed to disease, most notably tuberculosis, but the Publich Health Law of 1902 did nothing about these conditions.

The private practitioners of the Union movement saw many dangers in the public health movement. These practitioners successfully resisted the centralization of public health. They also refused to cooperate with programs which the practitioners believed would give the C.C.H.P. authority over medical practice. Doctors perceived the reporting of cases of contagious disease and of cause of death to be a threat to their clienteles. The Union tried to block legislation to enforce these measures and, when they failed, many doctors simply defied the law and refused to cooperate with the C.C.H.P. in tracking the course of contagious disease. Doctors also helped to cut back the dispensary movement in tuberculosis care, as the Lille case clearly indicates. Generally, the Union fought free care of any kind, including free vaccination and consultations in hospitals, unless the clientele was strictly limited.

Clearly the first three decades of the Third Republic were an era of critically important activity in medical politics. In this era, private practitioners were able to realize the affirmation of their vision of medical care. Although doctor-politicians at the department level did not always promote or share the goals of the Union, the Union still had great political influence in the national legislature and bureaucracy exercised through important doctor-politicians who were friends of the movement. Most important, however, was the seemingly unquestioned positive impact that, as an article of faith, so many politicians believed physicians had on society. Without truly examining the alternatives to private practice or its effectiveness, the legislature and public assistance bureaucaracy backed an expanded monopoly for private practitioners and passed laws which would help to increase their presence in society. This was the way in which the government chose to enact the socio-political concerns of solidarism. Better health and equality in medical care came to mean private practice as the principal form of medical care and often the only form of care available. In the course of these events, older collectivist forms of care were destroyed and a good deal of the new public health agenda was blocked.

BIBLIOGRAPHY

I. Archives and Government Publications

France. Archives nationales. AD XIX; F8 12, 168-174; F15 175, 178, 210, 239-241, 252, 3819, 4257-4261; F17 2292-2293; F22 520.

France. Chambre des Députés. *Journal Officiel* Meulan: Imprimerie nationale. 1892, 1893, 1898, 1902.

France. Conseil nationale de Recensement et Ecole des Hautes Etudes en Sciences sociales. *Paroisse et Communes de France, Dictionnaire d'histoire administrative* et démographique. Vols. 60, 62. 1974, 1975.

France. Institut national de la statistique. *L'Annuaire Statistique de la France.* 1878-1935.

France. Ministére de l'Intérieur. Direction de l'Assistance et de l'Hygiène publique. *Conseil supérieur de l'Assistance publique.* Fasicules 1-61. 1891-1910.

France. Ministére de l'Intérieur. Direction de l'Assistance et de l'Hygiène publique. *Récueil des Travaux de la Commission permanente de preservation* contre la tuberculose. Vols I-II. Paris: Imprimerie nationale. 1903-1907.

France. Ministére de l'Intérieur. Direction de l'Assistance et de l'Hygiène publique. *Récueil des Travaux du Comité consultatif d'hygiène publique.* Vols. I-XXX. Meulan: Imprimerie nationale, (1872-1902).

France. Ministére de l'Intérieur. Direction de l'Assistance et de l'Hygiène publique. Paul Roux et Henri Raynier. *Statistique sanitaire des Villes de France.* 1886-1905.

France. Ministre de la Santé. *Récueil des Textes officiels concernant la protection de la santé publique.* Vols. I-IX. Paris: Imprimerie nationale, 1957.

France. Ville de Paris. *Annuaire Statistique de la Ville de Paris.*

France. Ville de Paris. Préfecture de Police, Commissions d'hygïene de Département de la Seine, Rapports généraux. 1890-1892.

II. Contemporary Printed Sources.

Academie de Médecine. *Index biographique des membres, des associés et des correspondants de l'Academie de Médecine.* Paris: Doin, 1820-1970.

Alison, Dr. A. *Etiologie de la fièvre typhoide dans les campagnes.* Paris: Asselin et Cie., 1880.

_____ *Lettre à l'Academie sur l'épidémie actuelle de fièvre grippale a Baccarat en Juin 1890.* Paris: Asselin, 1890.

_____ *Memoire sur l'épidémie de grippe de 1891-92 dans la circonscription médicale de Baccarat.* Paris: V. Goupy et Jourdan, 1892.

_____ *Etude sur l'épidémie de Cholera qui a regne du 16 septembre au 6 décembre 1873 à Mervillei Canton de Baccarat.* Nancy: 1874.

Anquetin, N.P. *De l'Assistance publique et du service de santé dans les communes rurales.* Rouen: Cagniard, 1863.

Baudin, Léon. *L'Etat sanitaire, Besançon qu cours des derniéres années.* Besançon: Paul Jacquin, 1893.

_____ *Rapport sur un projet de creation d'un bureau d'hygïene. Besançon:* Paul Jacquin, 1889.

_____ *Ville de Besançon. Dix annés d'études démographiques et sanitaire (1888-98).* Besançon: Paul Jacquin, 1898.

Bertillon, Jacques. *La probĺeme de dépopulation.* Paris: A. Colin, 1897.

Bianchon, Horace. *Nos grandes Médecins d'Aujourd'hui.* Paris: Société d'éditions scientifique, 1891.

Bouvier, Jean. *Précis des lois d'assistance et d'hygïene publique.* Paris: 1807.

Brouardel, Paul. *Alimentation en eau de la Ville de Toulouse.* Paris: Bailliére, 1890.

_____ *Assainissement de Toulon.* Paris: Bailliére, 1885.

_____ *l'Exercise de la Médecine et le Charlatanisme.* Paris: Bailliére, 1899.

_____ *Des modes de propagation de la Fièvre typhoide. Conférence au Congrès, d'hygiène et de démographie de Vienne.* Paris: J.B. Bailliére et Fils, 1887.

_____ *La nouvelle loi sur la santé publique.* Paris: Bailliére, 1904.

_____ *La Profession médicale au commencement du XXe siècle.* Paris: J.B. Bailliére, 1903.

_____ *La Responsabilité médicale.* Paris: J.B. Bailliére et Fils, 1898.

_____ *Le Secret médical.* Paris: J.B. Bailliére, 1893.

Brouardel, Paul et P. Chantemesse. *Enquète sur les causes de l'épidémie de fièvre typhoide qui a regne à Clermont-Ferrand pendant les mois de Septembre, Octobre, Novembre 1886.* Paris: J.B. Bailliére et fils, 1887.

Brouardel, Paul et L.H. Thoinot. *La Fièvre typhoide.* Paris: J.B. Bailliére, 1895.

Chalot, Georges. *Les Bureaux d'hygiène en France (Paris et Seine excéptés).* Toulouse: Librarie Ch. Dirion, 1906.

Chevandier, Antoine Daniel. *Chambre des Députés. Proposition de loi relative aux enterrements civiles.* Paris: Quantin, 1880.

Commenge, O. *Les médecins des bureaux de bienfaisance et le nouveaux reglement du traitement à domicile.* Paris: 1889.

Coreil, M.F. *Rapport sur les travaux éffectivés par le Bureaux d'hygiène et le laboratoire municipale de Toulon 1904-1905.* Toulon: Direction du Bureau d'hygiène, 1905.

Constans, A., et A. Falliers. *Projet de loi sur l'assistance médicale gratuite.* Paris: 1890.

de Crisenoy, Jules. *Questions d'Assistance publique traitées dans les conseils genéraux.* Paris: 1888-1905.

Curzon. D. *Rapports sur l'organisation de la médecine rurale*. Nantes: Mellinet, 1846.

Dechambre, A. and L. Lerebouelet. *Dictionnaire encyclopedique des sciences médicales*. 1866-1889.

Duclaux, Emile. *L'hygiène sociale*. Paris: 1902.

Durand-Claye, A. *L'épidémie de Fièvre typhoide à Paris en 1882*. Paris: Etudes Statistique, 1882.

Fillassier, P. *De quelques causes de décès à Paris de 1893 à 1912*. Paris: Prefecture de la Seine, 1913.

Ichok, G. *Récueil des Textes officiels concernant la protection de la Santé publique*. Vol I-III. Paris: Ministre de la Santé, 1900.

Jaumés, Alphonse. *Le Déclaration des causes de décès et des malades épidémique*. Montpellier: C. Boohm, 1889.

Lésieur, Maurice. *Répertoire officiel de la Médecine et de la Pharmacie française*. Paris: 1896.

Martin, Andre Justin. *Essai d'organisation de la médecine publique en France*. Paris: Masson, 1880.

_____ *Commentaire admnistratif et technique de la loi du 15 fevrier 1902 relative à la protection de la santé publique*. Paris: Masson, 1905.

_____ *Des épidémies et des maladies transmissables dans leurs rapports avec les lois et reglements*. Lyon: Storck, 1889.

Mignot, A. *Topographie médicale de l'arrondissement de Gannat (Allier)*. Moulin: Congrès Scientific de France, 1870.

Napias, Henri. *L'Assistance publique dans le département de Saimbre-et-Loire*. Paris: Lecrosnier, 1890.

_____ *Rapport et projet de reglement pour l'application de la loi de juin, 1893*. Meulan: Imprimerie administratif, 1893.

Napias, Henri et A.J. Martin. *L'Etude et les progrés d'hygiène en France de 1878 à 1882*. Paris: G. Masson, 1882.

Pelloutier, F.M. *La Vie ouvrière en France*. Paris: 1900.

Proust, Adrien Achille. *L'Orientation nouvelle de la politique sanitaire*. Paris: Masson et Cie., 1896.

Réverchon, Louis. *Création d'un Bureau d'hygiène à Lyon*. Thèse, Lyon: 1882.

Trelat, Marcel. *Le loi du Fev. 1902 relative à la protection de la Santé publique. Ses consequences juridiques et pratiques dans les communes*. Paris: 1905.

III. Periodicals

Academie de Médecin, Commission permanente des épidémies, Rapports générals

Annales d'Hygiène publique, industrielle et sociale.

Annales d'hygiène publique et de médicine legale.

Bulletin de l'Academie de Médecine.

Bulletin officiel des Sociétés médicales des arrondissements de Paris et de la Seine.

Bulletin des Sociétés médicales d'Arrondissement et du Conseil général des Sociétés médicales du Département de la Seine.

Bulletin des Syndicat des médecins de France.

Bulletin des Syndicats médicaux du Nord et de Pas-de-Calais.

Bulletin du Syndicat médical de Lille et de la Région.

Bulletin officiel du Syndicat des médecins du Rhône.

Bulletin officiel de l'Union des Syndicats médicaux français.

Bulletin officiel du Syndicat des Médecins de la Seine

Bulletin de la Société de Médecine publique et d'Hygiène professionelle.

Bulletin de la Société de médecine de Bescancon.

Le Concours médical, Journal Hebd. des Médecins, Organe officiel de la Société professionnelle, "Le concours médical" et des Syndicats des Médecins de

France.

Le Courrier médical.

l'Echo médical de Lyon.

La France médicale et Paris médical.

La Fédération médicale du Sud-Ouest.

Gazette Hebdomadaire des Sciences médicales de Bordeaux.

Gazette des Hôpitaux.

Gazette médicale de Liège

Gazette médicale de Paris.

Journal de la société de statistique de Paris.

Lyon médical.

La Provence médicale.

Revue des Etablissements de bienfaisance et d'assistance.

Le Revue philanthropique, Revue d'Assistance, et Bulletin de la Société Internationale pour l'étude des questions d'assistance.

Revue d'hygiène et de Police sanitaire.

IV. Secondary Sources

Ackerknecht, Erwin H. *History and Geography of the Most Important Diseases.* New York: Hafner Co., Inc., 1965.

_____ "Hygiene in France, 1815-1848," *Bulletin of the History of Medicine,* V. 22, n. 2. (Mar.-Ap., 1948).

_____ *Medicine at the Paris Hospital 1794-1848.* Baltimore: John Hopkins Press, 1967.

_____ *A Short History of Medicine* Baltimore: John Hopkins Press, 1966.

Adams, T. "Moeurs et hygiène publique au XVIII siècle, Quelques aspects des dépôts de mendacité," *Annales de Démograhie Historique,* (1975).

Anderson, Robert David. *France, 1870-1914: Political and Society.* London: Routledge, 1977.

Aries, P. *Histoire des population français et de leur attitude devant la vie depuis le XVIII siècle.* Paris: Editions de Seuil, 1971.

Armengaud, André. "Avante Propos: Misére, Maladies et Assistance," *Annales du Midi,* V. 86. n. 199, (Oct.-Dec., 1974).

_____ "Quelques aspects de la pratique d'un médecin rural en Haute Languedoc au début de XX siècle," *Annales de Bretagne,* V. 86 N. 2 (June 1979).

_____ "Quelques Aspects de l'hygiène publique à Toulouse du XX siècle," *Annales de Démographie historique,* (1975), pp 131-137.

Aron, Jean-Paul, Jean-Pierre Goubert, and Jean-Pierre Peter, "La médecine et les médecins en France depuis deux siècles," *Annales de Démographie historique,* N. 11 (1974), pp 15-21.

Berlant, Jeffrey, *Profession and Monopoly.* Berkeley: University of California Press, 1975.

Biraben, J.N. "La Diffusion de la Vaccinations en France au XIX siècle," *Annales de Bretagne* V. 86, n. 2 (June 1979).

Boyer, Michel. "L'encadrement médical dans l'Ardèche du XIXe siècle," *Revue de Vivarais,* N. 653 (1978), pp. 16-31.

Brogan, Denis William. *The Development of Modern France,* V. 1 Westport Conn.: Greenwood Press, 1974.

Burnet, Macfarlane. *Natural History of Infectious Disease.* 2nd ed. Cambridge: Cambridge University Press, 1953.

Burrow, James G. "Organized Medicine," *Encyclopedia of Bioethics.* New York: Macmillan, 1978.

Cariage, J.L. *L'Exercise de la Médecine en France à la fin du XIX siècle.* Besançon: Impr. neotypo, 1965.

Chapman, Guy. *The Third Republic of France, the First Phase, 1871-1894.* New York: St. Martins Press, 1962.

Chastenet, Jacques. *Histoire de la Troisième République.* Paris: Hachette, 1974.

Chatelain, Able, "Valeur des récensements de la population française au 19e siècle," *La Revue de geographie de Lyon,* Vol. 29, (1954).

Coe, Rodney. *Sociology of Medicine.* New York: MacGraw Hill, 1978.

Coury, C.R. *L'Enseignement de la médecine en France, des orgines à nos jours.* Paris: Expansion scientifique français, 1968.

Derfler, Leslie. *Alexandre Millerand, The Socialist Years.* Paris: Mouton, 1977.

Donzelot, Jacques. *The Policing of Families.* with a foreward by Jacques Deleuze, trans. by Robert Harley. New York: Pantheon Books, 1979.

Dubois, René. *The Mirage of Health: Utopian Progress and Biological Change.* New York: Anchor Books, 1959.

Durey, Michael. *The Return of the Plague: British Society and the Cholera 1831-32.* Dublin: Gill and MacMillan, 1979.

Faure, Olivier. "Physicians in Lyon During the Nineteenth Century: An Extraordinary Social success," *Journal of Social History* V. 10, n. 4 (Summer, 1977).

Forrest, Alan. "Le Révolution et les hôpitaux dans le département de la Gironde," *Annales du Midi,* V. 86, n. 119 (Oct.-Dec. 1974).

Foucault, Michel. *The Birth of the Clinic.* trans. by Sheridan Smith. New York: Pantheon Books, 1973.

Freidson, Eliot. *Profession of Medicine, A Study of the Sociology of Applied Knowledge.* New York: Dodd, Mead and Company, 1970.

Gelfand, Toby. *Professionalizing Modern Medicine, Paris Surgeons and Medical Science and Institutions in the 18th Century.* Westport Conn.: Greenwood Press, 1980.

Goguel, Francois-Nyegaard. *La politique des partis sous la IIIe République.* Paris: Editions de Seuil, 1946.

Goubert, Pierre. *Sur la Population française au XVIII et XIX siècles*. Paris: Société de Démographie historique, 1973.

Goubert, Jean Pierre. "L'Art de Guerir. Médecine savante et médecine populaire dans la France de 1790," *Annales, Economies, Sociétés et Civilisations* (Sept-Oct, 1977). p 908.

_____ "Eaux publique et démograpie historique dans la France urbaine du XIX siècle, Le Cas de Rennes" *Annales de Démographie historique*, (1975).

_____ "The Extent of Medical Practise in France Around 1780," *Journal of Social History*, V. 10, n. 4 (Summer 1977), p. 410.

_____ *Malades et Médecins en Bretagne 1770-1790*. Paris: Klincksieck, 1974.

_____ "La pénétration du médecine dans le corps social en France, 1770-1850," *Histoire des Sciences médicales*, V. XIV, n. 4 (1980).

_____ "Reseau médical et médicalisation en France à la fin du XVIII siècle," *Annales de Bretagne*, V. 86, n. 2 (June 1979).

Gouldner, Alvin W. *The Coming Crisis of Western Sociology* New York: Avon Books, 1970.

Grmek, Mirko D. "Prélemenares d'une étude historique des maladies," *Annales, Economies, Sociétés, et Civilisations*. V. 24, n. 6 (Nov-Dec. 1969), p. 1473.

Guillaume, Pierre. "Malades, médecine et médecins à Bordeaux au XIXe siècle," *Annales de Bretagne*, V. 86, n. 2 (June 1979).

Hastings, Paul. *Medicine, An International History*. New York: Praeger, 1974.

Hatzfeld, Henri. *Le Grand Tournant de la médecine liberale*. Paris: Les Editions ouvriers, 1963.

_____ *Du Paupérisme à la Sécurité sociale* Paris: Librarie Armand Colin, 1971.

Hayward, J.E.S. "The Official Philosophy of the French Third Republic: Léon Bourgeois and Solidarism," *International Review of Social History*, V. 6 (1961).

_____ "Solidarism: The Social History of an Idea," *International Review of Social History*, V. 4 (1959).

Heller, Robert. "Officiers de santé, the Second Class Doctors of Nineteenth Century France," *Medical History,* V. 1, n. 22 (Jan. 1978).

Imhof, Arthur. "The Hospital in the Eighteenth Century for Whom?", *Journal of Social History,* V. 10, n. 4 (Summer, 1977).

Jacquement, Gerard. "Médecine et maladies populaires dans le Paris de la fin de XIXe siècle," *Recherches, l'Haleine des Faubourgs,* N. 29 (Dec. 1977), pp 245-283, 349-364.

_____ "Urbanisme parisien: la bataille du tout-à-l'égout à la fin du XIXe siècle", *Revue d'Histoire moderne,* V. 86 (Oct-Dec. 1979).

Knibiehler, Yvonne. "La Lutte anti-tuberculeuse, (1870-1930)," *Annales de Bretagne,* V. 86, n. 2.

de Kruif, Paul. *Microbe Hunters.* New York: Harcourt Brace and Co., 1926.

La Berge, Anne Fowler. "The French Public Health Movement," *Proceedings of the Western Society for French History,* V. 3 (1975).

_____ *Public Health in France and the French Public Health Movement* 1815-1948. Ph.D. Dissertation, University of Tennessee, 1974.

Larson, Magali Sarfatti. *The Rise of Professionalism.* Berkeley: University of California Press, 1977.

Lecuyer, Bernard-Pierre. "Démographie statistique et hygiène publique sous la monarchie censitaire," *Annales de Démographie historique,* (1977), pp 215-45.

_____ "Médecins et observateurs sociaux: Les Annales d'Hygiène publique et de Médecine légale (1820-1850)," *Pour une histoire de la statistique,* V. 1.

Lemay, Edna. "Thomas Herier, A Country Surgeon Outside Angouleme at the End of the 18th Century," *Journal of Social History,* V. 10, n. 4 (summer 1977).

Léonard, Jacques. "Les Débuts du 'Concours Médical'". *Histoire des Sciences médicales* V. XIV, n. 4 (1980).

_____. "Les Etudes médicales en France entre 1815-1848," *Revue d'Histoire moderne et Contemporaine,* V. 13 (Jan-Mars. 1966).

_____ *Les Médecins de l'Ouest au XIXe siècle,* Thèse de Doctorat d'Etat. Univ. de Paris (1976). Paris: Champion, 1978.

_____ *Les Officiers de Santé de la Marine française de 1814 à 1835.* Paris: Klincksieck, 1967.

_____ *La Vie quotidienne des médecins de province au XIXe siècle.* Paris : Hachette, 1977.

Léonard, Jacques, R. Darquenne, et L. Bergeron, "Médecins et Notables sous le Consultat et l'Empire," *Annales, Economies, Sociétés, et Civilisations* V. 32, N. 5 (Sept.-Oct., 1977).

McInnes, Mary Elizabeth. *Essential of Communicable Disease.* St. Louis: C.V. Mosley, 1975.

McKeown, Thomas. "Fertility, Mortality and Causes of Death, An Examnation of Issues Related to the Modern Rise of Population," *Population Studies* V. 32 (1978), p 535.

_____ *Medicine in Modern Society.* London: Oxford University Press, 1965.

_____ *The Modern Rise of Population* London: Edward Arnold, Ltd., 1976.

McKeown, Thomas and thomas McLachlan. *Medical History and Medical Care.* London: Oxford University Press, 1971.

McKeown, Thomas and R.G. Record. "Reasons for the Decline of Mortality in England and Wales During the Nineteenth Century," *Population Studies,* XVI (1962-63), p 94. Mayeur, Jean-Marie. *Débuts de la Troisième République, 1871-1898.* Paris: Editions de Seuil, 1973.

Mitchell, Barbara. *French Revolutionary Syndicalism: A Study in Pragmatic Revolt.* Ph.D. Dissertation, University of California, Riverside, 1982.

Mitchell, Harvey. "Rationality and Control in French Eighteenth Century Medical Views of the Peasantry," *Comparative Studies in Society and History,* V. 21, N. 1 (June 1979), p 82.

Noland, Aaron. *The Founding of the French Socialist Party (1893-1905).*

Parsons, Talcott. "The Professions and Social Structure," *Essays in Sociological Theory,* 1954.

_____ "Social change and Medical Organization in the United States. A Sociological Perspective," *The Annals of the American Academy of Political and Social Science,* N. 346, (March 1963).

Pernick, Martin S. "Medical Professionalism," *Encyclopedia of Bioethics.* New York: Macmillan. 1978.

Prevost, M. and Roman d'Amat. *Dictionaire de Biographie française.* Paris: Librarie Letouzey, 1956.

Ramsey, Matthew. "Medical Power and Popular Medicine: Illegal Healers in 19th Century France," *Journal of Social History,* V. 10, n. 4 (Summer 1977).

Rosen, George. "Historical Trends and Future Prospects in Public Health," *Medical History and Medical Care,* Thomas McKeown and Thomas McLachlan eds. London: Oxford Univ. Press, 1971.

_____ *A History of Public Health,* 1958.

Rosenberg, Charles S. *The Cholera Years, The United States in 1832, 1849 and 1866.* Chicago: University of Chicago Press, 1962.

Shyrock, Richard. *The Development of Modern Medicine, An Interpretation of the Social* and Scientific Factors Involved. New York: Alfred A. Knopf, 1947.

_____ *The Development of Modern Medicine.* Madison: University of Wisconsin Press, 1979.

Spengler, Joseph. *France Faces Depopulation.* Durham, S.C.: Duke University Press, 1938.

Stage, Sarah. *Female Complaints, Lydia Pinkham and the business of Women's Medicine.* New York: W.W. Norton, 1979.

Sussman, George D. "Enlightened Health Reform, Professional Medicine and Traditional Society: The Cantonal Physicians of the Bas-Rhin, 1810-1870," *Bulletin of the History of Medicine,* V. 51, n. 4 (1977).

_____ *From Yellow Fever to Cholera. A Study of French Government Policy,* Medical Professionalism and Popular Movements in the Epidemic Crises of the Restoration and the July Monarchy. Ph.D. Dissertation, Yale University, 1971.

_____ "The Glut of Doctors in Nineteenth Century France," *Comparative Studies in Society and History*, V. 19, n. 3 (July, 1977).

Swart, Koenraad. *The Sense of Decadence in Nineteenth Century France*. The Hague: Nijhoff, 1964.

Thuiller, Guy. *Histoire de l'Administration français au XIX siècle*. Paris: Annals Ecole des hautes Etudes en Science sociale, 1976-77.

_____ "Pour une histoire régionale de léau, en Nivernais au XIX siècle," *Annales, Economies, Sociétés, et Civilisations* V. 23, n. 1 (Jan-Fev. 1968).

_____ "Pour une histoire de l'hygiène coporelle un exemple régional, le Nivernais," *Revue d'histoire économique et sociale* (1968).

Varagnac, Andre. *Civilisation traditionelle et genres de Vie*. Paris: Albin Michel, 1948.

Vess, David M. *The Medical Revolution in France, 1789-1796*. Gainesville: Florida State University Press, 1975.

Weber, Eugen. *Peasants into Frenchmen, The Modernization of Rural France, 1870-1914*. Palo Alto: Stanford University Press, 1976.

Weisz, George. "The politics of Medical Professionalization in France 1845-1848," *Journal of Social History*, V. 12, n. 1 (Fall 1978).

Wood, W. Barry. *From Miasmas to Molecules*, New York: Columbia University Press, 1961.

Youngson, A.J. *The Scientific Revolution in Victorian Medicine*. New York: Holmes and Meier, 1979.

Zeldin, Theodore. *France, 1848-1948, Vol. I., Ambition, Love and Politics*. London: Oxford University Press, 1973.

APPENDIX I

FUNCTIONING OF MEDICAL ASSISTANCE PROGRAMS
1887(1)

I.A
THE FUNCTIONING OF MEDICAL ASSISTANCE PROGRAMS
IN DEPARTMENTS UNDER THE LANDAIS SYSTEM
IN 1887

Departments	Percent Indigents Eligible	Percent Indigents Treated(2)	Expenses Per Indigent Treated
Allier	1.6	26.9	38.49 francs
Indre	2.0	26.9	10.31
Ardennes	3.9	30.6	11.21
Indre-et-Loire	4.7	19.8	12.66
	3.0	26.1	18.17

---

1. C.S.A.P., Fasc. 9, Tableaux I and II. Calculations were done using SPSS on a Prime Computer at the Lab for Historical Research, University of California, Riverside. Figures presented here are roundoff to one decimal place and totals may not agree due to round off error.
2. Measured as a percent of indigents eligible.

I.B
THE FUNCTIONING OF MEDICAL ASSISTANCE PROGRAMS IN DEPARTMENTS UNDER THE CANTONAL SYSTEM
1887

Departments	Percent Indigents Eligible	Percent Indigents Treated	Expenses Per Indigent Treated
Bouches-du-Rhône	3.2	27.0	11.58 francs
Nièvre	1.4	42.5	14.52
Basses-Alpes	3.7	34.5	18.27
Meuse	4.2	25.3	23.97
Aude	2.9	49.8	8.47
Tarn	4.0	26.3	8.12
Haut-Rhin	6.1	52.7	7.25
Ariège	7.1	29.6	5.62
Hérault	5.5	36.1	4.68
Hautes-Alpes	12.1	23.7	5.16
Isére	5.3	16.2	10.10
Haute-Garonne	3.9	27.6	7.01
Meurthe-et-Moselle	7.3	15.8	9.66
Somme	10.3	16.2	10.05
Loiret	4.9	29.8	7.88
Deux-Sevres	4.0	33.8	5.90
Drôme	3.0	58.5	4.40
Loire	5.7	24.8	4.68
Basses-Pyrenées	8.1	44.8	7.17
Maine-et-Loire	4.9	52.1	9.90
Ille-et-Vilaine	10.3	33.0	3.45
Pas-de-Calais	14.8	34.5	5.78
	6.0	33.4	8.8

I.C

THE FUNCTIONING OF MEDICAL ASSISTANCE PROGRAM
IN DEPARTMENTS UNDER MIXED SYSTEMS
1887

Departments	Percent Indigents Eligible	Percent Indigents Treated	Expenses Per Indigent Treated
Landes	3.7	35.8	12.68 francs
Seine-et-Oise	2.9	55.1	22.64
Saône-et-Loire	2.9	25.9	16.29
Vaucluse	5.1	37.6	10.05
Tarn-et-Garonne	5.2	43.1	11.54
Haute-Saône	6.5	61.5	48.30
Gers	3.2	36.2	10.74
	4.2	42.2	18.89

I.D

THE FUNCTIONING OF MEDICAL ASSISTANCE PROGRAMS
IN ALL DEPARTMENTS
1887

Percent Indigents Eligible	Percent Indigents Treated	Expenses Per Indigent Treated
5.3	34.3	12.07

APPENDIX II
FUNCTIONING OF MEDICAL ASSISTANCE PROGRAMS
1899(1)

II.A
FUNCTIONING OF MEDICAL ASSISTANCE PROGRAMS
IN DEPARTMENTS UNDER LANDAIS SYSTEMS
1899

Departments	Percent Indigents Eligible(2)	Percent Indigents Treated(2)	Expenses Per Indigent Treated(4)	Percent Indigents Hospital-ized(5)
Ain	2.4	24.0	17.5 francs	3.8
Allier	2.7	31.0	15.5	1.8
Ardèche	3.4	20.2	10.9	1.9
Ardennes	1.9	38.5	26.7	2.7
Aveyron	6.3	33.8	9.5	0.9
Bouches-du-Rhône	1.8	41.1	18.6	1.2
Calvados	6.6	16.6	16.7	1.7
Cantal	3.3	30.2	22.2	1.5
Charente	3.5	26.3	19.3	3.0
Charente-Inférieure	2.8	46.3	17.1	
Côte'd'Or	3.0	19.4	13.7	2.4
Côtes-du-Nord	4.1	19.6	23.1	2.5
Creuse	1.2	43.0	20.4	1.2
Dordogne	3.2	32.4	13.6	1.2
Finistére	6.4	25.5	9.9	1.9
Gard	1.5	23.3	19.6	3.2
Haute-Garonne	7.3	49.0	16.1	1.1

1. C.S.A.P., Fasc. 92, Tableaux I, II, IX. See footnote 1, Appendix I for information on calculations.
2. Indigents listed as eligible under the program, measured is a percentage of the participating population.
3. Indigents treated under home care programs, measured as a percentage of the indigent enlisted as eligible.
4. Expenses under home care per indigents treated under home care.
5. Indigents hospitalized, measured as a percentage of indigents enlisted.

II.A
FUNCTIONING OF MEDICAL ASSISTANCE PROGRAMS
IN DEPARTMENTS UNDER LANDAIS SYSTEMS
1899 (CONTINUED)

Departments	Percent Indigents Eligible	Percent Indigents Treated	Expenses Per Indigent Treated	Percent Indigents Hospitalized
Gers	2.6	70.0	10.6	0.5
Gironde	2.2	51.9	21.2	6.1
Indre	4.1	77.1	6.5	1.9
Indre-et-Loire	6.4	21.9	13.0	1.5
Jura	5.2	25.1	17.3	0.8
Loir-et-Cher	4.6	29.8	16.4	2.1
Haute-Loire	2.4	24.3	17.4	2.3
Loire-Inférieure	3.7	36.7	11.2	0.4
Lozére	5.8	25.3	22.4	2.3
Maine-et-Loire	4.6	30.8	12.3	1.9
Manche	5.7	10.2	28.4	0.8
Marne	2.0	31.2	22.3	3.9
Haute-Marne	2.0	32.3	8.9	1.8
Mayenne	7.0	28.4	6.4	0.8
Nièvre	4.4	32.6	14.9	2.6
Orne	2.5	24.1	9.5	1.5
Puy-de-Dôme	3.4	40.3	17.8	
Basses-Pyrenées	5.4	45.2	8.8	
Savoie	4.2	21.3	13.6	4.1
Seine-Inférieure	9.8	26.1	20.1	1.8
Seine-et-Marne	4.8	30.1	23.4	1.8
Tarn	3.1	39.4	9.0	0.9
Var	1.1	49.5	27.4	5.2
Vaucluse	4.8	36.9	13.8	1.6
Vendée	2.5	38.5	14.5	1.0
Vienne	3.2	40.4	15.6	1.9
Haute-Vienne	2.0	43.8	18.2	5.1
Vosges	5.6	14.9	13.2	0.4
Yonne	2.4	36.8	20.8	2.9
	3.9	33.3	16.2	2.1

II.B
FUNCTIONING OF MEDICAL ASSISTANCE PROGRAMS
IN DEPARTMENTS UNDER CIRCUMSCRIPTION (CANTONAL) SYSTEMS
1899

Departments	Percent Indigents Eligible	Percent Indigents Treated	Expenses Per Indigent Treated	Percent Indigents Hospitalized
Aisne	6.3	27.2	13.3 francs	3.9
Ariège	7.0	99.7	4.3	0.3
Corrèze	6.5	38.0	9.2	1.1
Doubs	3.0	19.6	30.6	1.5
Ille-et-Vilaine	11.2	32.9	5.8	1.1
Isére	5.6	56.0	5.9	1.8
Meurthe-et-Moselle	4.2	23.3	15.2	4.5
Meuse	3.5	27.6	12.7	0.4
Pas-de-Calais	12.1	38.9	6.8	
Pyrenées-Orientales	1.5	7.7	39.6	4.8
Haut-Rhin (Belfort)	3.0	62.3	14.1	0.2
Sarthe	9.6	32.2	7.4	1.6
Deux-Sevres	9.6	14.3	14.6	0.5
	6.4	36.9	13.8	1.8

II.C
FUNCTIONING OF MEDICAL ASSISTANCE PROGRAMS
IN DEPARTMENTS UNDER MIXED SYSTEMS
1899

Departments	Percent Indigents Eligible	Percent Indigents Treated	Expenses Per Indigent Treated	Percent Indigents Hospitalized
Basses-Alpes	2.9	33.4	18.7 francs	2.2
Hautes-Alpes	7.7	25.2	13.4	1.7
Aube	2.8	34.5	12.7	2.3
Aude	7.3	42.7	23.1	1.6
Cher	4.5	32.7	12.1	
Corse	5.3	39.2	15.6	0.6
Drôme	3.6	28.7	20.3	4.5
Eure	3.9	45.9	17.2	2.8

II.C
FUNCTIONING OF MEDICAL ASSISTANCE PROGRAMS
IN DEPARTMENTS UNDER MIXED SYSTEMS
1899 (CONTINUED)

Departments	Percent Indigents Eligible	Percent Indigents Treated	Expenses Per Indigent Treated	Percent Indigents Hospitalized
Eure-et-Loir	5.0	45.6	14.3	3.1
Hérault	5.0	24.6	21.1	3.3
Loire	4.5	31.4	13.3	4.5
Loiret	6.9	36.5	12.9	2.3
Lot	10.5	37.1	9.7	0.7
Nord	13.2	37.1	8.2	0.6
Oise	8.3	19.2	21.8	1.2
Hautes-Pyrenées	5.2	0.7	41.1	0.8
Rhône	2.3	23.5	21.8	0.2
Haute-Saône	6.0	12.1	42.4	0.5
Saône-et-Loire	3.3	27.3	12.7	3.1
Haute-Savoie	5.2	15.8	12.9	1.6
Seine-et-Oise	2.1	99.0	3.0	12.6
Somme	4.8	23.0	6.9	
Tarn-et-Garonne	5.3	45.4	14.6	1.4
	5.4	37.3	17.0	2.5

II.D
THE FUNCTIONING OF MEDICAL ASSISTANCE PROGRAMS
IN ALL DEPARTMENTS
1899

Percent Indigents Eligible	Percent Indigents Treated	Expenses Per Indigent Treated	Percent Indigents Hospitalized
4.7	29.3	16.0 francs	2.1